Decolonised and Developmental Social Work

T0179110

This is the first book to cover existing debates on decolonising and developmental social work whilst equipping readers with the understanding of how to translate the idea of decolonisation of social work into practice. Using new empirical data and an extensive detail of social, cultural, and political dimensions of Nepal, the author proposes a new model of 'decolonised and developmental social work' that can be applicable to a wide range of countries and cultures.

By using interviews with Nepali social workers, this text goes beyond mere theoretical approaches and uniquely positions itself in a way that embraces rigorous bottom-up, grounded theory method. It will further ongoing debates on globalisation-localisation, universalisation-contextualisation, outsider-insider perspectives, neoliberal-rights and justice oriented social work, and above all, colonisation-decolonisation of social work knowledge and practice. It also promotes solidarity of, and the struggle for, progress for those in the margins of Western social work and development narrative through an emerging theory-praxis of decolonised and developmental social work.

Decolonised and Developmental Social Work is essential reading for students, academics, and researchers of social work and development studies, as well as those striving for a decolonial worldview.

Raj Yadav, PhD, is from Nepal, and now makes his temporary home in Australia. His interest lies in decolonising epistemologies and their use in advancing knowledge production in the fields of social work and development. He has worked as a lecturer and has contributed to social work curriculum development in universities in Nepal and Australia.

Indigenous and Environmental Social Work Series
Series Editor: Hilary Weaver
University at Buffalo, USA

Sustainability is the social justice issue of the century. This series adopts a global and interdisciplinary approach to explore the impact of the harmful relationship between humans and the environment in relation to social work practice and theory. It offers cutting-edge analysis, pioneering case studies and current theoretical perspectives concerning the examination and treatment of social justice issues created by a disregard for non-Western cultures and environmental detachment. These books will be invaluable to students, researchers, and practitioners in a world where environmental exploitation and an ignorance of indigenous peoples is violating the principles of social justice.

Titles:

Decolonised and Developmental Social Work
A Model From Nepal
Raj Yadav

For a full list of titles in this series, please visit: www.routledge.com/Indigenous-and-Environmental-Social-Work/book-series/IESW

Decolonised and Developmental Social Work

A Model From Nepal

Raj Yadav

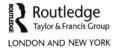
Routledge
Taylor & Francis Group

LONDON AND NEW YORK

First published 2019
by Routledge
2 Park Square, Milton Park, Abingdon, Oxon OX14 4RN

and by Routledge
52 Vanderbilt Avenue, New York, NY 10017

First issued in paperback 2020

Routledge is an imprint of the Taylor & Francis Group, an informa business

British Library Cataloguing-in-Publication Data
A catalogue record for this book is available from the British Library

Library of Congress Cataloging-in-Publication Data
A catalog record for this book has been requested

ISBN 13: 978-0-367-67147-1 (pbk)
ISBN 13: 978-1-138-33344-4 (hbk)

Typeset in Bembo
by Apex CoVantage, LLC

Contents

Figures

Tables

Abbreviations

AFU	Agriculture and Forestry University
AIN	Association of International NGOs
APASWE	Asia-Pacific Association of Social Work Education
BSW	Bachelor of Social Work
CBO	Community-based organisation
CHHE	Caste Hill Hindu Elite, includes Brahmin, Kshatriya (or Chhetri), Thakuri, and Dashnamis
DIMM	*Dalits, Indigenous (or Janajatis), Madheshis*, Muslims
FWU	Far-Western University
GO	Government organisation
GoN	Government of Nepal
HO	Humanitarian organisation
IASSW	International Association for Schools of Social Work
ICSW	International Council on Social Welfare
IFSW	International Federation of Social Workers
INGO	International non-governmental organisation
LBU	Lumbini Bauddha University
MDGs	Millennium Development Goals
MWU	Mid-Western University
MSW	Master of Social Work
NCP	Nepali Congress Party
NGO	Non-governmental organisation
NGSDO	Non-government Social Developmental Organisation
NPC	National Planning Commission
NSU	Nepal Sanskrit University
PoKU	Pokhara University
PRSP	Poverty Reduction Strategy Paper
PU	Purwanchal University
SDC	Social Development Council
SPA	Seven Parties Alliance
SWC	Social Welfare Council
TU	Tribhuvan University
UNDP	United Nations Development Program
VDC	Village development committee

Acknowledgements

Though I am the author of this book, I would be arrogant in claiming that all the ideas contained herein, and thus the result – this book – is my own. With the support of many people, I have continuously used reflective reading and critical reasoning to study, analyse, and reference diverse scholarly works to build upon prior ideas in structuring my arguments for this book. I owe a debt of gratitude to the scholars who have blazed pathways in this endeavour. I also wish to recognise the following:

This journey would not have been easy without:

Mel Gray

I accomplished this goal with the support of:

Kylie Agllias and Amanda Howard

And I thank those who dared to raise their voices and think differently:

The participants in Nepal

For enriching my thinking about decolonised and developmental social work:

Mel Gray, Michael Yellow Bird, John Coates, James Midgley, and Ibrahim A. Ragab, only to name a few here

And for bringing this work forward:

All the folks at Routledge including Georgia Priestley and Nick Craggs

People who stood by me:

Benjaporn Meeprom, Soobhiraj Bungsraz, Rohith Thota, Justin Nicolas, and Amit Kumar Yadav

For unconditional love:

My parents, brothers, and sister

Notes on transliteration and Nepali terminology

In this book, 'Nepal' refers to the 'Federal Democratic Republic of Nepal', which was called the 'Kingdom of Nepal' until the monarchical rule of the Shah Dynasty ended on May 28, 2008. Up until the 20th century, 'Nepal' referred to the Kathmandu Valley, while the country was called 'Gorkha'.

I have consciously used the term 'Nepali' rather than its variant 'Nepalese'. The term 'Nepalese' does not belong to the Nepali vernacular. Rather, it is the product of the Anglicisation of Nepal and gained popularity among elite English-speaking Nepali people, expats, and Western tourists. The term 'Nepali', used in this book, refers generally to the diverse peoples of Nepal and anything pertaining to them, such as language, culture, costume, lifestyle, values, and norms. Nepal is a pluralist society and the use of 'Nepali' conveys its diversity and heterogeneity.

It is easy to pronounce Nepali terms, as there is no contradiction between the script and pronunciation of the words as used in day-to-day life. However, there are some exceptions, especially the letter *'V'*, which is pronounced *'B'*, for instance, in the word *'vikash'*. Likewise, instead of flapping the tongue, the sound *'Chh'* comes from the throat, such as used in the word *'Chhaupadi'*. The sound *'Th'* is tricky as *'h'* may be aspirated, such as in *'Kathmandu'*, or non-aspirated, such as in *'sanstha'*. Also, one would notice that each Nepali word has a consonant or consonant unit and a vowel used alternatively, for instance, *'bideshi'* appears as b (consonant), i (vowel), d (consonant), e (vowel), sh (consonant unit), and i (vowel) (Shrestha & Bhattrai, 2017).

Meaning of Nepali terms and cultural practices

Atithi devo bhava – a guest is equivalent to God

Badi communities – are traditionally untouchable caste group and often engaged in commercial sex work despite its illegal status in the country

Bahudal – multiparty democracy system after 1990

Bhumi Puja – is a Hindu ritual performed to worship the earth

Bideshi sanstha – refers to organisations working in Nepali territory with their roots outside of the country

Bideshi siksha – means education that has foreign influence

Bideshi vikash – literally means 'foreign development'; *bideshi* is 'foreign' in the Nepali language. When coupled with *vikash* (development), it typically refers to 'development initiated outside' or 'development initiated by outsiders'. In general, Nepali peoples refer to INGO-led development as *bideshi vikash*

Bihe – marriage

Bistarai – slowly, as in *bistarai basnus* (sit slowly), *bistarai janus* (travel slowly), *bistrai khanus* (eat slowly), and *bistarai garnus* (perform slowly)

Bhoj-Bhatera – feast

Chhaupadi Pratha – is a Hindu caste groups' custom of Western Nepal, which holds that women are impure at the time of menstruation. Women are required to live in a shed rather than the main dwelling when they are menstruating. Despite outlawed by the government in 2017, *Chhaupadi Pratha* continues even today

Dana – charity

Dharma – religion; in Hindu society, it is believed that *dharma* and *karma* lead a person toward *moksha*, that is, salvation

Dharm bhakari – local grain bank

Dhikur – is the organisational concept of saving and credit

Guthi – is trust; it refers to a clan or caste-based informal religious, social, or cultural organisation

Haina ra – is a sort of tag question, used in day-to-day conversation to affirm certain things, arguments, or claims

Hajur – means yes, which sometimes also conveys second person personal pronoun used to respect elders

Hariyo ban Nepal ko dhan – greener forest is Nepal's wealth

Janajati – is a local word for Indigenous People

Karma – fate or duty (it is our fate in life to do our duty)

Kot Parva – refers to the coup of 1846 orchestrated by Rana to curtail then monarch's power. It resulted into 104 years autocratic Rana regime

Kshama Puja – is a Hindu ritual carried out for pardon from a god

Kuwa – a well

Madhesh Aandolan – refers to *Madheshis* people's protests for inclusion in the mainstream politics

Malami – mourning

Moksha – salvation

Nwaran – celebration of the ninth day of birth

Padhera – learning through formal education

Pahade and Madhishe – refers to the people living in the hills and lowlands of Nepal, respectively. They are sometimes associated with caste and linguistic groups. For instance, a caste group speaking the Nepali language but living in the lowlands might not introduce him or herself as *Madhishe* but will feel proud to be *Pahade*

Panchayat – a community level institution active to facilitate local affairs during *Panchayat* system

Panchayat system – a partyless system under the direct rule of the monarch between 1960 and 1990

Parera – learning through experience

Parma – labour exchange system

Pati-pauwa – shelter

Paropkar – voluntary service

Samajik karya – voluntary activity

Samajik nyay – social justice

Samajik Sewa Ain – Social Service National Co-ordination Act

Samanta – equality

Sewa – an act of selfless service, which is also used interchangeably with *paropkar*

Siyos – suffix used in ex-royal's day-to-day communication

Sukila mukila pesha – the phrase *sukila mukila* is linked to *Prachanda* – the chair of the Maoist Party of Nepal. By using this terminology, he symbolically meant bourgeois class of the society. When combined with the word *pesha* – profession, this refers to the profession of bourgeois class

Swadeshi aadhar – domestic foundation for something, such as development

Swadeshi abdharna – refers to national or domestic vision

Tapai – second person personal pronoun used to respect elders

Teej – festival celebrated mainly by CHHE women to ensure their husbands' longevity and prosperity

Terai – lowland, also known as *Madhesh* in day-to-day communication

Vikashi kura – literally means 'development debate'

Vandevta – god of the forest

Vasudhaiva kuṭumbakam – the world is one family

Foreword

The discourse on decolonisation is relatively new to social work and social work has yet to explore the decolonisation literature found in the social and political science disciplines. A key issue for decolonisation scholars is naming by outsiders. Hence, in this welcome addition to the literature on international social work, Raj Yadav clarifies his stance at the outset:

> I have consciously used the term 'Nepali' rather than its variant 'Nepalese'. The term 'Nepalese' does not belong to the Nepali vernacular. Rather, it is the product of the Anglicisation of Nepal and gained popularity among elite English-speaking Nepali people, expats, and Western tourists. The term 'Nepali', used in this book, refers generally to the diverse peoples of Nepal and anything pertaining to them, such as language, culture, costume, lifestyle, values, and norms. Nepal is a pluralist society and the use of 'Nepali' conveys its diversity and heterogeneity.
> (see 'Notes on Translitarian and Nepali Terminology' – in this book)

Raj continues in this vein to demonstrate his incisive understanding of the political, cultural, and social history of Nepal and the various changes that have occurred over time, as well as the social relationships between classes and ethnic groups that divide its society. In describing and analysing the sociocultural groups of Nepal, he demonstrates the complexities of the caste system and the cleavages, conflicts, and new politics shaping contemporary Nepali society in which social work is seeking to find its place. Through his empirical work, he aptly shows why we need to be cautious in reading prior work on social work's development in Nepal and provides the first critical reading of the dynamics surrounding an occupation that has yet to achieve professional and social legitimacy. To date, social work in Nepal is an educational enterprise training graduates for non-existent jobs, a situation that revels all the ethical and political complexities of social work's internationalising ambitions. The sociopolitical complexities of the Nepali landscape highlight the over-ambitious claims of social work's international definition that presumes a fit-for-purpose too difficult to reach in many countries in the Global South. What better place to start such a critical examination than with those few social workers, relative to the number who have graduated from Nepal's social work education programs over the last three decades, working in the field of social development. Raj's focus on evolving development practice among social workers working in INGOs enabled him to ask important question about the relevance of

Nepal's growing social work education enterprise. As he explores their experiences, he learns of the problems of imported social work and the mountain practitioners have to climb to fashion culturally appropriate and contextually situated responses in Nepal. It is they, rather than their social work educators, who are carving out a place for social work in this complex sociopolitical terrain. Drawn by his critical curiosity, Raj bravely questions the relevance of Western social work to the Nepali context, seeking to discern from practitioners in the development field what social work education and practice tailored to fit this context might look like. His book offers an incisive exposition, based on empirical research, of what home-grown social work in Nepal might entail.

For Raj, locally relevant social work responsive to the complex Nepali socioeconomic, political, and cultural context has much to gain from a decolonised model of practice in which Nepali social workers exercise their right to determine for themselves forms of practice responsive to local needs, rather than the interests of dominant international and regional social work organisations seeking to promote a universal notion of professional social work. Thus, Raj juxtaposes the situation of social work in Nepal and its colonial origins against a critique of western social work, in the process aligning it with indigenous and decolonising social work models. By taking an inductive, bottom-up, grounded theory approach to explore the nature, principles, and practice imperatives emerging from within Nepal, Raj finds incontrovertible evidence of what home-grown Nepali social work might involve. In this way, he enables social workers employed in INGOs, whom he regards as knowledge keepers and co-constructors of reality, to share their lived experience and thus contribute to a decolonised and developmental model of Nepali social work. By situating this exploration in the historical context, he provides a sound argument for the need to transform social work education, policy, practice, and research across Nepal. He uses his personal and professional insights and positionality to further nuance his empirical exploration in a meaningful way, demonstrating his genuine commitment to decolonising Nepali social work. By grounding his arguments in social workers' experiences of programs endeavouring to respond to localised and regional needs, and micro, mezzo, and macro issues, he highlights the holistic nature of decolonised and developmental social work. As Raj himself writes,

> 'Decolonised, developmental Nepali social work' reflects Nepali social workers' creative energy in advocating an emancipatory mindset and interjecting greater autonomy, self-determination, and responsiveness to local social, cultural, and political dynamics. The social work participants in this book collectively define development in terms of the needs of the Nepali population and view 'Nepalisation' as a right of Nepali social workers to honour the dignity and worth of Nepal's multilingual and multiethnic populations with whom they work. . . . The resultant model of 'decolonised, developmental Nepali social work' is thus unique to Nepal, a country that continues to negotiate the contemporary phase of sociocultural and political transition, yet enshrines a fresh notion of decolonisation coupled with development from which many like-minded social workers across the globe might draw meaning in their contexts.
>
> (see the Preface of this book)

Raj offers a case study worthy of emulation. This book, then, provides a useful resource to those striving to decolonise social work education, policy, practice, and research across the immediate region and more broadly. Its insights on the pitfalls of colonising

influences should make social workers wary of the damage they do when they intervene in international contexts foreign to them leaving locals to make sense of what
they have left behind. We need to ask ourselves whether we want to make social work
an undoing project. In a sense this is what Raj and the social workers in his study were
seeking to do to fashion meaningful social work practice for a small, landlocked country
in the Global South.

Mel Gray

Preface

In this book, I examine evolving social work practice in Nepal among those working in international non-government organisations (INGOs). It explores the extent to which Nepali social workers, employed in INGOs, perceive the relevance of their social work education to practice. It seeks their views on culturally appropriate and contextually situated social work in Nepal. In brief, this book examines what social work education and practice tailored to the Nepali context might look like based on the assumption that social work should be responsive to the socioeconomic, political, and cultural context in which it is practised. Given the paucity of knowledge about the practice of social work in Nepal, this book has used a grounded theory approach to examine the perceived synergy between social work education and the practice of social work as it is emerging in INGOs. The resultant model of 'decolonised, developmental Nepali social work' reflects the contemporary narratives of social workers engaged in the development activities of INGOs in Nepal. While international and global stakeholders insist on the universalisation and globalisation of social work, this work details how, in the mid-1990s, a small landlocked nation, sandwiched between two giant superpowers, India and China, had Western social work thrust upon it, and how some social work graduates have been crafting a unique decolonised and development based social work model in their day-to-day practice. Their narratives affirm that the uncritical importation of Western social work has resulted in disillusionment among Nepali social workers, due to the tensions between their Western-styled educational training and the competing and complex sociocultural and political processes of Nepali society. These social workers, who I have interviewed for this book, also claim that the 'Nepalisation' of social work will entail an incremental building-block approach to decolonisation.

The systematic process in this book involves the integration of local Nepali world views in the social work and development discourses, a process that is far less glamourous than those writing enthusiastically about the global movement of social work will have us to believe. In this way, the 'Nepalisation' of social work will have a permanent legacy of questioning the importation of social work into Nepal. The coming decades will act as a corrective to social work's historical role in Nepal's ongoing tumultuous history as Nepali social workers use their cultural and symbolic values, draw on their strengths and social capital, and transform borrowed Western social work to fit local fields and spaces.

'Decolonised, developmental Nepali social work' reflects Nepali social workers' creative energy in advocating an emancipatory mindset and interjecting greater autonomy, self-determination, and responsiveness to local social, cultural, and political dynamics.

The social work participants in this book collectively define development in terms of the needs of the Nepali population and view 'Nepalisation' as a right of Nepali social workers to honour the dignity and worth of Nepal's multilingual and multiethnic populations with whom they work.

Using constructivist grounded theory within qualitative research, this book allows the narrative of 'decolonised, developmental Nepali social work' to emerge from social workers at the coalface, while blending my interpretation as an author to yield a co-constructed decolonised and developmental model for social work practice in Nepal. The key argument of this book has been developed against the backdrop of divergent debates on globalisation-localisation, universalisation-contextualisation, outsider-insider perspectives, heteronomy-sovereignty, neoliberal capitalism-rights and justice-oriented social work, and above all, the colonisation-decolonisation of social work knowledge and practice. This has led to a model responsive to local sociocultural traditions (cultural focus), power and structural dynamics (structural focus), Nepali problems and issues (contextual focus), and poverty (development focus). The resultant model of 'decolonised, developmental Nepali social work' is thus unique to Nepal, a country that continues to negotiate the contemporary phase of sociocultural and political transition, yet enshrines a fresh notion of decolonisation coupled with development from which many like-minded social workers across the globe might draw meaning in their contexts.

Prologue

An honest, heretofore untold story of Nepali social work

Not only was the last decade of the 20th century the most vibrant in Nepal, with expectations of transformation in the state and polity running high, but it was also the most important in Nepal's history, as the Nepali people's long struggle for democracy materialised into a multiparty democratic system of governance ending an era of authoritarian rule in 1990. Between 1990 and 1995, none of the three prime ministers, who served the cabinet, completed their five-year tenure and 1996 was an especially important year, first because the tenuous coalition government of the Nepali Congress Party (NCP), Rastriya Prajatantra Party, and Sadbhawana Party was struggling to sustain the emerging democracy under Prime Minister Sher Bahadur Deuba. This shaky coalition government faced immense challenges, not only from the highly polarised political parties keeping his tenuous administration together, but also due to the corruption and fiscal indiscipline that prevailed at that time (Hachhethu, 1997). Thus, the fledgling democracy, with its populist slogans of liberalisation, decentralisation, and governmental reform, was overshadowed by the coalition government's simultaneous making and unmaking of politics (Pfaff-Czarnecka, 2004a).

Second, as if this were not enough, the Maoist insurgency, inspired by its blend of Leninist, Marxism, and Maoism ideologies, began the so-called People's War, which encircled the cities from the countryside in 1996. The decade-long insurgency caused the death of about 15,000 Nepali people, while many were displaced or disappeared. The Nepali Maoists planned to complete

> the new democratic revolution after the destruction of feudalism and imperialism . . . then immediately moving toward socialism, and, by way of cultural revolutions based on the theory of continuous revolution under the dictatorship of the proletariat, marching to communism – the golden future of the whole humanity.
> (Communist Party of Nepal, Maoist, 1995, n.p.)

They claimed that, through armed struggle, they would free Nepal from its petty bourgeois, narrow nationalist, religious-communalist, and caste-based illusions.

Third, when Father Charles Law, a Chicago-based Jesuit missionary, introduced social work education at St Xavier's College in Kathmandu in 1996, the Nepali polity was still struggling to sustain its fledgling multiparty democracy, on the one hand, and to understand the guerrilla uprising, on the other. Earlier, in 1987, fellow missionary, Brother James F. Gates, had introduced Western-style social work training at the Social Work Institute (SWI) in Kathmandu. Contrary to Nepali macro-structural conditions, this new technology of service delivery and management envisaged a role for social work, as a profession with a social mission based on individualistic Western models. Its hidden agenda was to commemorate and continue the unfinished legacy of Saint Francis Xavier's (1506–1552) Christian expansionist mission to East and South Asia.

These missionaries introduced social work into Nepal as a modern, scientific project based mainly in psychological models. The education program they introduced targeted young peoples, mainly in the capital city of Kathmandu, and linked them physically through social work institutes, ideologically through Western concepts, and technologically through universal skills and techniques. The landscape of this new idea allowed previously disconnected Nepali youth to think and act homogeneously by introducing them to Western texts, concepts, and, above all, the idea of cultural production. Its English language lent common terminologies of doing service that had no equivalents in Nepali languages. Despite all these, it failed in overall to encourage a critical engagement with Nepal's multilinguistic, multicultural, and multiethnic populations. One of the dubious contributions of the Western missionaries, or colonisers in general, to Nepal was that they introduced colonial concepts, the English language, and rational models. They also aided international aid agencies that shaped non-government services in Nepal. An elite group of social work educators readily adopted the Western social work brand and embraced its fundamental tenets. For me, the driving question is, 'Are Nepali social workers happy with this?'

Chapter 1

Thinking about decolonised and developmental social work

With its introduction by Western missionaries three decades ago, about 50 private colleges affiliated to four Nepali universities, mainly in the capital city of Kathmandu, teach social work in Nepal. Until now, there have not been any empirical studies to examine the relationship between social work education and practice in Nepal. Essentially, the primary stakeholders driving social work education are educational institutions, educators, and practitioners, motivated by the belief that social work can play a vital role in enhancing Nepal's development into a fully fledged democracy. However, in the absence of a service infrastructure employing social work graduates, there is little knowledge about the organisational settings in which they are employed, though most willing to have employment opportunity in INGOs. Given this backdrop, this book critically examines evolving Nepali social work practice among those working in INGOs of Nepal. It also explores the extent to which Nepali social workers, employed in INGOs, perceive their social work education to be relevant to their practice. It seeks their views on culturally appropriate and contextually situated social work in Nepal.

Drawing on its epistemology from post-colonial studies in general and recently emerging decolonising discourse within social work in particular, the book has emerged out of my doctoral degree and has its inception in my long-standing critical thinking and questioning about the fit of Western social work to a non-Western context like Nepal. In other words, the book explores the home-grown nature of social work based on the advocacy that social work should be responsive to the socioeconomic, political, and cultural context in which it is practised. This book uses a bottom-up approach to examine the perceived synergy between social work education and the practice of social work as it is emerging through INGOs in Nepal. In so doing, the book empirically responds to, *inter alia*, how relevant is the imported social work education to the work of Nepali social workers employed in INGOs; does the education Nepali social workers receive indeed have a Western bent, and, if so, how does it prepare Nepali social workers for the situations they encounter in their day-to-day practice; do Nepali social workers share ongoing concerns on the need to decolonise and shift towards developmental social work in Nepal, and, if yes, what might a model of decolonised and developmental social work practice look like in Nepal?

Why decolonised and developmental social work?

As the central theme of this book, I wondered whether 'decolonisation' was the correct term to use in relation to a country like Nepal, which had never been formally colonised by external forces. Initial forays into the literature on decolonisation affirmed this choice since 'maritime enclaves' and 'settlement colonies' were not the only manifestations of colonisation. It existed where exploitation and 'quasi-colonial control', 'informal rule', and even 'non-colonial determinant influences' (Jürgen, 1997, pp. 21–22) prevailed. The decolonisation discourse polarised the West and non-West. Al-I Ahmad (2004) believed,

> There is not only a great gap between the two groups, but . . . an unfillable chasm deepening and widening by the day. Thus, wealth and poverty, power and incompetence, knowledge and ignorance, prosperity and ruin, civilization and savagery, have been polarized in the world. One pole is held by the sated – the wealthy, the powerful, the maker and exporters of manufactures. The other pole is left to the hungry – the poor, the impotent, the importers and consumers, . . . The difference arises not just from the time and place – it is not just a quantitative one. It is also qualitative, with two diverging poles: on the one hand, a world with its forward momentum grown terrifying and, on the other, a world that has yet to find a channel to guide its scattered motive forces.
>
> (p. 58)

For decolonisation scholars, Western missionaries introduced their cultural and religious values while running rough shod over traditional cultures and social support networks that had long sustained Indigenous Peoples in the colonies they sought to transform to Western world views. Colonial aggressors pursued their territorial agenda through war and violence, if necessary, to claim supremacy over, and bring modernisation and enlightenment to, so-called 'uncivilised people'. Thus, the missionaries who brought social work education to Nepal colonised young Nepali minds introducing a profession based on Western ways of thinking and doing, undergirded by Western values. This continues in Nepal's educational institutions that teach social work. These concerns led to my interest in studying the 'decolonisation' of social work in Nepal.

Development is another key theme alongside decolonisation in this book that warrant explanation from the outset. As discussed in-depth later in Chapter 3 and Chapter 6, thinking about Nepali social work within the developmental purview is two-fold. First, as Murdie (2014) suggested, development as the need for Nepali population delivers human security that

> is recognised as coming both from freedoms that protect citizens from state repression and political violence and from the overall material well-being of the country. Many of those outcomes can be couched in language concerning the promotion of economic, social, and cultural rights (freedom from want) outlined in the Universal Declaration of Human Rights . . . and in outcomes listed as political and civil rights (freedom from fear).
>
> (p. 29)

Thus, developmental social work with a focus on human security model is best suited to address the needs of Nepal given its state of underdevelopment. As explained in Chapter 6, the integration of development into decolonising social work emphasises a rights-based notion of community development approach to deal with the issues of

> deprivation [that] remains a key aspect of life in Nepal. More than eleven million people – nearly half of its population – live below the poverty line and almost 38

percent live below $US 1 per day. There are growing inequities between rural and urban areas, and substantial discrimination against women, *Dalits* and indigenous minorities persists.

(Kernot, 2006, p. 298)

On the other, in its second aim, developmental focus of Nepali social work encompasses a critical view of development that goes beyond the concept of 'pathological misdevelopment' (Ingram, 2018, p. 110) often touted in international development discourse. Instead, it embraces post-development perspective to view development itself as an imported entity in Nepal and, therefore, promotes the notion that development perspective should be guided by the notion of 'self-expression' and 'self-determination' as several post-development theorists (for example, Fujikura, 2001; Pigg, 1992, 1993; Shrestha, 1997) have argued in the case of Nepali development.

Decolonised and developmental social work: pedagogy, politics, and praxis

The social reconstructionist traditions have made several proposals to counter the challenges of ongoing hegemonic and colonial effects in social work. Most of them have evolved around the notion of culture and its variants such as cultural competence, cultural sensitive, cultural appropriateness, and cross-cultural, only to name few here. Rather situating the term decolonisation in the epistemic and existential context of struggles in which social work 'leaders and peoples mutual identified, together create the directive lines of their action' (Freire, 1974, p. 183) – educational, developmental, political, and liberation; these scholarships have provided a descriptive mode through writings in the hope that these will create patterns that might yield prescriptive norms in order to reverse the effects of West-centric social work in the 'Other' contexts. The failure to address political injustice in social work as well as in some occasions within the decolonisation debate and their tendency to enforce narrow indigeneity and cultural identities demand a critical alternative, one that re-thinks the 'Other' context by re-centering differences through a focus on the particularities of 'Others' mutual interdependence rather than generalities of 'Others' universality. Such thinking, according to Gaztambide-Fernández (2012) requires

on the one hand, a recognition of how social constructed categories of . . . [geographic, linguistic, and cultural variations within the national boundary, and likewise caste] and ethnicity, gender and sexuality, and social class have real and directive consequences on both the material and symbolic conditions that affect individuals and groups. On the other, it requires acknowledging that the consequences of such conditions are not always predictable and that particular circumstances and relationships enable or disallow particular responses and modes of being-with-others and acting in the world.

(p. 44)

Therefore, it is important that I outline the pedagogy and its politics and praxis from the very beginning that inspire the thinking about decolonised and developmental Nepali social work. Embedded in the critical, emancipatory notion of social work currently in vogue, the idea of decolonised and developmental Nepali social work rests on the decolonising pedagogy of solidary progress. More specifically, I argue that the decolonising pedagogy of solidary progress as introduced in this book is a conceptually dynamic worldview informed by a theoretical heteroglossia. In its conceptual dynamic sense, it draws on the constant tension arising from paradoxical process of globalisation, universalisation, internationalisation, and indigenisation and localisation debate in social work, whereas, in terms of theoretical heteroglossia, it has its inception in the works of post-colonial studies (Gandhi, 1998: Spivak, 1999), critical race theory (DuBois, 1961; Fanon, 1986), critical (decolonising) pedagogy (Gaztambide-Fernández, 2012; Mignolo, 2012), spatial theory (Soja, 1989), and active decolonisation in social work (Gray, Coates, Yellow Bird, & Hetherington, 2013a). Similar to what Yellow Bird (2013) has argued in general, the pedagogy of decolonising solidary progress goes beyond the blaming games such that first and foremost it ensures solidarity of Nepali peoples and simultaneously advocates frontline social workers to engage in achieving anticolonial, anti-racist, antisexist, anti-oppressive, antidiscriminatory, including anticasteism and antiethnocentrism, social work education and practice.

In other words, the decolonising pedagogy of solidary progress evokes a post-perspective in social work to unmask the ongoing insidious effects of domination, exploitation, oppression, and injustice all too visible in the importation of West-centric social work in 'Other' contexts. Within its post-perspective claim, or say simply as a post-social work perspective, it asserts the view that peoples in the 'Other' contexts who are the victims of Western enlightenment and modernist social work as well as West-centric development discourse must emphasise cultural-historical activity of solidarity to achieve progressive home-grown social work to ensure sustainable human development goals. Here, then in post-social work, the subaltern can speak to gain control over social work in their context. Borrowing from McLaren (1988), the decolonising pedagogy of solidary progress is thus 'irrevocably committed to the side of the oppressed' (p. 164) that equips social workers with the notion of rights-based developmental goals to ensure peoples' freedom from fear and want. The following are the positions that inform the conception of the pedagogy of solidary progress:

- Social work education and practice in 'Other' context should be understood in terms of 'West' versus 'rest of the West' and its related colonial and imperial links.
- Social work education and practice theories should encourage social work educators and students to engage and develop a critical understanding of the relationship among culture, ideology, and power.
- Social work education and practice is the subject matter of subjectivity that involves the context and its complexities, contradictions, contesting norms and values, and multiple realities.
- Social work process and practice must involve historical background as well the existing social, cultural, political, and developmental dynamics of the particular context.
- Social work education and practice should be analysed to understand the ways it primarily serves the interests of the wealthy and powerful urban classes while working in the name of poor, marginalised, and minorities.
- The relationship between social workers (as educators, students, practitioners, researchers, policymakers, advocate, and so forth) and peoples should be based on critical engagement and dialogue than merely objectifying the peoples as consumers, customers, or clients.

- Social work education and practice should engage in empowering marginalised and minorities sections of society and contribute to the emancipatory and developmental goals.
- Social work education and practice should focus on empowering 'self' prior to the mastery of professional and technical skills.
- Social work education and practice should be mindful to the modernist notion of objectivist inquiry and truth, and therefore should challenge the ongoing efforts for universalisation and globalisation of social work.
- And, above all, social work education and practice should bring peoples together in solidarity for their collective progress.

These positionalities bring us to the fore to view pedagogy as an intrinsic part of political nature of social work, which 'encompasses both an anticolonial and decolonizing notion of pedagogy and an anticolonial and decolonizing pedagogical praxis' (Tejeda, Espinoza, & Gutierrez, 2003, p. 18). Further, in its political sense, social work itself is the site for critical consciousness and activity where there is a need that adherents of decolonising discourse create solidarity to counter and eventually end the effects of colonisation that has sustained until now in social work. This way, the political notion promotes self-determination not only to re-design social work but also to re-envision and re-shape social work such that human development goals become central to social work interventions in 'Other' context.

In exploration about social work's political nature, it is also important to briefly highlight the diffusion of social work from the 'West' to the 'rest of West' and the ways this technological transfer has both distorted 'Others' day-to-day realities and silenced contextual voices. The pious motherhood and apple pie image of West-centric social work, to borrow from Munck (1999), continues to justify the West-centric social work image as faithful angel and places it as uncontested, universal human good (Specht & Courtney, 1994). Similar to what Esteva (1992) argued to critique development, the metaphor of social work 'gave global hegemony to a purely Western genealogy of history, robbing peoples of different cultures [in "Other" context] of the opportunity to define the forms of their social life' (p. 9). Social work's technological transfer advocated, and to an extent continues to do so even today, that one true path to civilisation and salvation as well as helping individuals, families, groups, and communities irrespective of varied contexts is to follow Western fashion of social work bent on 'capitalism, social Darwinism, the Protestant ethic and individualism' (Nagpaul, 1993, p. 214). The West is best, and the rest has to conform to it – social work's technological transfer explicitly preaches across the world. If there is world views, approaches, or intervention frameworks that do not result from Western social work genealogy, then those, no matters how effective they can be for local peoples, cannot be accommodated in or accredited as social work. The tragedy is that peoples everywhere, including in Nepal, have caught up in a Western perception of social work reality not realising that they have become an object for Western social work. The political goal within pedagogy of solidary progress is to unmask these dominant views and reinsert the home-grown perspectives of 'Other' and those who have been victims of these narratives. In essence, the political nature of pedagogy considers the experiences of 'Othering' as a point of departure where the subaltern, more specifically Nepali social workers, can speak and eschew 'double-consciousness' (DuBois, 1961), 'double-bind' (Spivak, 1999), or 'corporeal malediction' (Fanon, 1986).

In relation to decolonising social work, the pedagogy of solidary progress is not only about entering into theoretical discourse – creating another jargon that might only fit into academic debate. But, it is also about translating pedagogy into praxis that concerns how social work's imported Western root in 'Other' context can be altered on the one hand as well as can be used to reshape social work that genuinely provides social workers 'with a rich theoretical, analytical, and pragmatic toolkit for individual and social transformation' (Tejeda et al., 2003, p. 31) on the other. The transformative issues particularly in relation to Nepal concerns delivering rights and justice based developmental goals such that Nepali marginalised and minorities groups can become the part of mainstream Nepali society (see Chapter 2 and Chapter 6). In this sense, the idea of solidary progress as a praxis, or more specifically, solidary progress as a manifestation of conscientisation, resistance, and transformation, equips Nepali social workers with an inward-looking ability to compare between imported social work and what is needed on the grassroot levels.

Background to, and rationale for, the decolonised and developmental social work in Nepal

Figure 1.1 illustrates my conceptualisation of the diffusion of social work from its international centres in the USA and UK and its reinforcement via regional and international social work organisations, such as the Asia-Pacific Association of Social Work Education (APASWE), the International Federation of Social Workers (IFSW), and the International Association for Schools of Social Work (IASSW). It shows Nepal as a satellite of their influence, on the one hand, with India on the other, as the ensuing discussion shows.

Satellite connections: Western cuisine with an Indian flavour

The Jesuit missionaries introduced the Western invention of social work (Gray, Coates, & Yellow Bird, 2008a) from its colonial centre in the USA, along with US social work literature with its heavy psychological base in clinical, mental health. In the process of introducing social work education to Nepal, they relied on a neighbouring satellite, India, where social work, long established in the main urban centres, was not yet a recognised profession. They drew technical support from the social work institute, Nirmala Niketan, based in Mumbai (Nikku, 2010a). Thus, social work in Nepal resulted from the missionaries' Western colonial influence combined with Indian support. India had been colonised by Britain from 1858 to 1947, with Western social work introduced as part of the colonial welfare administration in 1936.

Indian social work remained steeped in Western influences, when, in 1996, Jesuit missionaries invited its social work academics in Nirmala Niketan to support its development in Kathmandu. Hence, Nepali social work might be described as a menu of 'Western cuisine with an Indian flavour'. The effects of what became the dominant satellite of India were present until recently in the two social work institutes in Nepal. Indian nationalities have run and managed St Xavier's College and the Nepal School of Social Work (joint initiatives of Kadambari Memorial College of Science and Management and Nepal College of Development Studies), which had laid the early foundations of social work education. They influenced curriculum development at the Bachelor and Master levels and represented Nepal in international and regional social work forums and organisations (Nikku, 2010a, 2010b; Nikku, Udas, & Adhikari, 2014).

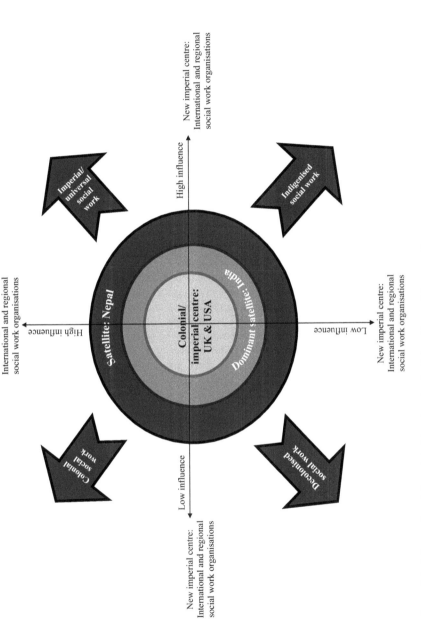

Figure 1.1 Advent of social work in Nepal and colonial and imperial connections

New imperial centres: regional and international and social work organisations

Despite ongoing resistance, new imperial centres in international and regional social work organisations have sought to institutionalise and legitimise Western social work's universalising, globalising, and internationalising agenda across the world (Gray et al., 2008a; Gray & Webb, 2014). Nepal is one of the centres vigorously pursued and supported in the Asia-Pacific Region (Nikku et al., 2014). Critics have referred to this territorialising agenda variously as 'colonising', 'westernising', 'globalising', 'Americanising', 'homogenising', 'imperialising', 'McDonaldising', and 'neoliberal fantasising' (Gray et al., 2008a; Harris & Chou, 2001; James, 2004; Midgley, 2008; Pugh & Gould, 2000; Webb, 2003). Gray and Webb (2014) believed international and regional social work organisations' efforts to legitimise their global agenda presented it as a benign influence. It invited the members of these international and regional organisations to act as forces of moral good, spreading social work education to new sites, while overlooking the political nature of this agenda and its injurious results in non-Western contexts. Here indigenous, culturally and ethnically sensitive, and decolonising social work practice were called for.

These professional social work organisations began to exert their influence in earnest in Nepal in 2005 (Nikku et al., 2014), despite critiques of social work's lack of fit with Nepal's 'feudalistic social structure framed in traditionalism . . . and institutions of self-help, and self-reliance' (Shrestha & Bhattrai, 2017, pp. 2–3). Not only were professional services foreign to Nepali culture, but also there was no word in any Nepali language and dialect to describe imported social work itself. Nevertheless, 'Western cuisine and Indian flavoured' social work education was introduced to Nepal, though it was offered mainly in Kathmandu. Social work remains an unknown entity outside this urban enclave, while a home-grown model of Nepali social work education and practice has yet to emerge. In short, given there is no welfare infrastructure to employ graduate social workers, there is no Nepali social work practice of which to speak. Further, local social workers have little knowledge of international social work structures and organisations. This was shown at the time of the 2015 earthquake, when I was interviewing Nepali social workers for this book. Most social workers on the ground were oblivious to the short-term, 'do-good' approach of the IASSW and the interventions or changes claimed in reports, forums, and electronic media from its allied international partners (IASSW, International Council on Social Welfare [ICSW], & IFSW, 2016; Nikku, 2015). Gray and Yadav (2015) have argued that international social work bodies were oblivious to Nepal's contemporary challenges, such as migrant workers, human trafficking, and military personnel returning from service without benefits, noting the

> need to take account of structural factors and political forces at work there. A privatized market-oriented, neoliberal agenda, totalitarian political parties, and donor-driven development are fundamental to the Nepal[i] nation state. Moreover, Nepal[i] development issues and policies are increasingly marked by transnational processes. Given the nation's complex sociopolitical circumstances, trapped as it is in vicious cycles of damaging internal problems, such as . . . struggling to find its way into legitimate policy, failed development, persistent poverty, lack of protection for minority rights, and centralized government, Nepal[i] social

workers face major challenge, and could do well with . . . [locally developed, home-grown models].

(p. 29)

Gray and Yadav (2015) further argued,

> Social work's international organizations, like all INGOs, promote . . . vested interests and events playing out in 'our own backyards' do not necessarily accord with the profession's humanistic and emancipatory agenda. Consequently, local contexts, cultures, problems, and practices are undermined under the frame of international social work organization's extreme penchant for universalizing social work.

(p. 28)

Four quadrants: possible influences and competing tensions

Against this backdrop, Figure 1.1 illustrates the possible influences on, and competing tensions in, Nepali social work shown in four quadrants:

> *Quadrant 1: Colonial social work*, that is, the high influence of international social work organisations versus the low effects of regional social work organisations.
> *Quadrant 2: Imperial-universal social work*, that is, the high influence of international and regional social work organisations.
> *Quadrant 3: Indigenised social work*, that is, the high influence of regional social work versus the low influence of international social work.
> *Quadrant 4: Decolonised social work*, that is, the low influence of international and regional social work organisations.

One example of colonial, imperial, and universal social work is evident in the literature. Then member representing Nepal on international and regional social work bodies, an Indian academic, has defined what a social worker in Nepal is as follows:

> 'Social Worker' in the context of Nepal refers to new graduates and current practitioners (both Nepalese and other nationals) with recognized social work qualifications, that is, Degree in Social Work [Bachelor of Social Work (BSW) or Master of Social Work (MSW)] or a Graduate Diploma in Social Work or a recognised Social Work qualification. These qualifications should be recognized or acceptable to associations like the Singapore Association of Social Workers and or International Association of Schools of Social work (IASSW).

(Nikku, 2014, p. 103)

In distinguishing social workers from frontline development workers without social work degrees, Nikku (2014) echoed the professional extremism of colonial and imperial social work. Calling social workers social service practitioners, he mirrored the distinction in the South African hierarchy of welfare personnel (Gray, 2000). He described them thus:

> Social Service Practitioners' are those who are working in the capacity of social workers performing social work functions for the major part of their work but are

without relevant social work qualifications like BSW and MSW. Executive directors, program executives, youth workers, field social workers, case workers, who are not formally trained in social work per se are performing social work functions for the major part of their work can qualify to be accredited as Social Service Practitioners if they meet the entry requirements for Social Service Practitioners. They can become accredited Social Workers if they go on to acquire a recognized Social Work qualification and also fulfil the other entry requirements for accreditation.

(Nikku, 2014, p. 104)

This distinction has been presented in the international social work literature and on international platforms at seminars, workshops, conferences, and meetings of international bodies. Both attempts and advocacies have been conducted to sanction this categorisation of Nepali so-called social service personnel without any formal input from, or consultation with, Nepali social workers. This has provoked several critical concerns and raised questions as follows:

- Are the international and regional social work organisations genuinely concerned about developing home-grown Nepali social work models to address ongoing structural chaos in Nepal?
- On what basis can 'other nationals' become spokespeople on, or adjudicators of, Nepali social work?
- Are social work's international and regional organisations legitimising universal social work by failing to consider local contingencies?
- Why should the Singapore Association of Social Work and, likewise, the IASSW be arbiters of what constitutes a social worker in Nepal, especially since, to the best of my knowledge, most social work graduates and Nepali social work institutes are oblivious to these international and regional social work bodies and their 'self-imposed' regional outsiders?
- Is Nepali social work an unfinished project of Western organisations and their professionalising, universalising mindset?
- Can Nepali social workers' rights to self-determination be promoted so they decide on their own version of social work depending upon the local needs of Nepali society rather than the dominance of international and regional social work organisations?

Despite such critical concerns, as a representative of IASSW and APASWE in the past, Nikku (2014) argued that 'regional organizations such as APASWE can play an important role in strengthening social work education in South Asian regions' (p. 107), including in Nepal. He ignored criticisms of indigenising processes following 'hard on the heels of social work's colonizing past and continue[s] its penchant for spreading itself with missionary zeal' (Gray & Coates, 2008, p. 13). Quadrant 3 represents indigenised social work, where there is high influence of regional social work and low influence of international social work forces (as shown in Figure 1.1). Others have been equally vocal in their criticisms of indigenisation for the following reasons:

- Indigenisation has promoted the burgeoning globalisation agenda and liberal utopian politics.

(Webb, 2003)

- Indigenisation has legitimised international and global social work.
  (Evetts, 1998)

- Instead of focusing on people-centred social work practice, indigenisation has championed international and global social work's universal values and standards.
  (Gray & Coates, 2008)

- Indigenisation has promoted contested world views of a common and shared professional identity on the one hand and transcending context on the other.
  (McDonald, Harris, & Wintersteen, 2003)

- Indigenisation does not challenge the professional managerialism and bureaucratism of Western social work. Under a professionalised ethos, it is difficult for frontline workers to deliver on the need for human rights and social justice.
  (Carniol, 2005)

Against this backdrop, what Nepali social work requires is Quadrant 4 – decolonised and developmental social work, where the influence of international and regional social work organisations is low (as shown in Figure 1.1). An emergent and alternative, decolonised and developmental Nepali social work would not only resist international and regional social work organisations' imperialist and universalist gaze, but also free itself from the grip of missionary-styled colonial social work. Contrary to the one-size-fits-all approach of global and universal social work, decolonised and developmental Nepali social work would seek to comprehend Nepali pluralist social structures, interactions, and norms and, thus, design social work interventions in a way that addresses contemporary macrolevel social, cultural, economic, and political issues. Decolonised and developmental social work would also reflect Nepali social workers' right to self-determination and deconstruct imported Western social work, which is out of step with Nepali society.

Genesis, central arguments, and inquiry method of the book

The genesis of this book is rooted in a transitional phase in my life, when I was about to begin a career in academia in Nepal after I had successfully completed a BSW in Nepal in 2007 and an MSW in India in 2010. I had accepted a full-time lecturing position at a private social work institute run by missionaries, while simultaneously working part-time at several other schools of social work in Nepal. My brief career as a young lecturer found me uncomfortable with an educational system based on Western models of social work and I began to explore how Jesuit missionaries had embedded Western social work education in Nepal, questioning its fit with Nepal's diverse social, cultural, and political traditions. This led to my interest in formulating a home-grown practice model to decolonise social work in Nepal.

Embarking on PhD study meant finding an appropriate empirical method with which to study my area of interest. Given my journey to that point, I was drawn to indigenous and decolonising views on social work and knowledge production. More than whimsy, a genuine concern for local knowledge production and my sense of insider responsibility encouraged me to embark on decolonisation of social work in Nepal through a PhD and then converting my thesis into this book. Nevertheless, living on the other side of the world (termed the Third World), I was oblivious to the ongoing debates and dialogues in indigenous and decolonising social work that had already got foothold among scholars in Australia, Canada, and the countries of Africa. Also, systematic qualitative inquiry and its world views, traditions, and approaches were something that I was encountering for the first time in my life. In other words, this was as much a journey about myself moving from a state of unknowing to knowing.

In addition, despite the need for decolonised and developmental social work in Nepal, awareness of this topic has yet to be felt in private discussions and public forums. Most importantly, due to the weak research base of social work training and practice, systematic knowledge production on decolonised and developmental Nepali social work has yet to emerge, not only in Nepal, but also in similar contexts, where literature is lacking on empirical and substantive, or middle-range, theories or models of decolonising social work. In recent years, however, debates on decolonising social work have increased piecemeal (Briskman, 2008; Gray, Coates, Yellow Bird, & Hetherington, 2013c; Gray & Hetherington, 2013; Harris, 2006; Rao, 2013; Sinclair, 2004; Tamburro, 2013; Waterfall, 2008; Yellow Bird, 2008).

Therefore, in this book I explore how a distinctly Nepali social work practice approach has been developing through examining the daily activities of social workers employed in INGOs in Nepal. I also explore, among other things, the extent to which local social workers question the relevance of the Western models they have learnt in relation to the sociocultural and structural constraints of Nepali society. Above all, with its focus on Nepali sociopolitical issues, I emphasise the political nature of social work in Nepal and the degree of political awareness attached to the roles Nepali social workers play in the country. In other words, in this book I aim to explore and document the features and principles of a distinctive Nepali social work practice approach. Thus, the book set forth with the following objectives:

1   To critically examine colonialism as the major root of professional social work and its resultant impact in Nepal.
2   To explore social work practice in relation to broader Nepali social, economic, cultural, and political frameworks and service-delivery mechanisms.
3   To identify processes underway, and barriers to, the decolonisation of social work practice in Nepal.
4   To develop a model of social work practice in Nepal, which is distinctly local and well-integrated with the Nepali sociostructural environment.

To accomplish these objectives, I examine what the 'Nepalisation' of social work model framed in a localised, context-specific way might entail (Guba & Lincoln, 1985; Lofland & Lofland, 1995). I embrace an inductive, bottom-up, grounded theory approach to explore the nature, principles, and practice imperatives emerging from within Nepal and to discern what a home-grown Nepali social work model might involve (Charmaz, 2006; Glaser & Strauss, 1967; Strauss & Corbin, 1990). Worth noting here, the book involves Nepali social workers (see Table 1.1) employed in INGOs as knowledge keepers or co-constructors of reality rather than mere participants in, or objects of, the model introduced in this book (Berger & Luckmann, 1966) and rigorously explores their lived experience of Nepali social work (Seidman, 2013) 'to discover what is going on [in Nepali social work], rather than assuming what should go on' (Glaser, 1978, p. 159). Their direct and lived experiences have been synthesised to a model decolonised and developmental Nepali social work and extensively discussed in Chapter 7.

Table 1.1 Characteristics of research participants

Participants*	Age	Gender	Qualification	Working areas
Kiran	26	Male	BSW	Children
Namita	28	Female	MSW	Community development
Niharika	24	Female	BSW	Children
Niti	30	Female	BSW	Community development
Ranjan	32	Male	BSW	Children
Ritesh	33	Male	BSW	Peacebuilding/conflict management
Samikshya	31	Female	BSW, MSW	Community development
Sujit	32	Male	BSW	Community development
Tulshi	34	Female	MSW	Children
Urmila	32	Female	BSW, MSW	Community development
Total n = 10, female = 6, male = 4				

*Not their given names

In an exploration, after carefully assessing the existing methodological choices, I employ a grounded theory method, which seems to fit with the decolonising ontological, epistemological, and axiological stance and the aims of the book, as it offers a culturally safe and respectful way of exploring Nepali social work (Rigney, 1999). In particular, the book utilises a concept of the constructivist grounded theory that emphasises the co-construction of knowledge (Charmaz, 2006; Dei & Johal, 2005). The heart of grounded theory lies in its inductive method, whereby knowers theorise from their interactions in their real world. This seemed to cohere with my own intuition that Nepali social work needs to respond to national and local issues. Moreover, the use of grounded theory method in the book also holds the promise in reducing the gap between Western theory – the *status quo* – and Nepali social workers' on-the-ground experience. For Glaser and Strauss (1967), generating a bottom-up theory, or a model in the case of this book, involves a process of knowledge production in which the knowledge production cannot be divorced from systematic data collection, multiple levels of data analysis, and early stage constant comparisons. Here was a way to address the mismatch between imported Western and locally grounded Nepali social work. Glaser and Strauss's (1967) grounded theory sought a 'fit' between the research or knowledge production and the context in which its findings would be implemented. In Strauss and Corbin's (1990) systematic grounded theory, 'data collection, analysis, and theory stand in reciprocal relationship with each other' (p. 23). And, above all Charmaz's (2006) constructivist grounded theory that informs the enquiry method for this book emphasised the co-construction of knowledge. These all epistemologically and ethically suit the book's goals of understanding the multilayered social situation and realities of Nepali social workers who have been regarded as active actors in 'Nepalisation' of social work. Thus, this book has chosen a constructivist grounded theory approach (Charmaz, 1995a, 2000, 2006, 2009, 2011) to model the concept of decolonised and developmental Nepali social work for the following reasons:

• It allows exploration of its subject matter through a focus on the complex social and personal forces that shape individual lives and begins where practitioners are.

Its inductive nature 'typically invites the reader into vicarious experience and therefore, is positioned to give voice to the voiceless'.

(Gilgun, 2011, pp. 346–354)

- It reshapes the interaction between knower and knowledge keepers in the process of knowledge production and equips the knower as the 'author of a reconstruction of experience and meaning'.

(Mills, Bonner, & Francis, 2006, p. 2)

- It assumes that the interaction between knower and knowledge keepers 'produces the data, and therefore the meanings that the . . . [knower] observes and defines'.

(Charmaz, 1995b, p. 35)

- It positions the knower as a co-producer of knowledge and allows him or her to add 'a description of the situation, the interaction, the person's affect and perception of how the' making sense goes.

(Charmaz, 1995b, p. 33)

- The knower's voice does not transcend the experience of the knowledge keepers but re-envisages it bringing 'fragments of fieldwork time, context, and mood together in a colloquy of the author's [or knower's] several selves – reflecting witnessing, wondering, accepting – all at once'.

(Charmaz & Mitchell, 1996, p. 299)

The exploratory nature of this book on a topic about which little is known in Nepal demands a reflexivity to make sense of Nepali social workers' worldview. Again, the key aim of the book is to explore what Nepali social work practice entails through an examination of what social work practitioners in INGOs are doing daily in Nepal. This leads to the formulation of 'grand-tour' questions, such as, are they aware of the wider sociostructural context of their work? Do they ask questions about how the work they are doing is contributing to social change? In so doing, how do they question the relevance of the social work education program they have received in preparing them for practice in Nepal? To this end, the key questions that guide this book are:

- To what extent do Western ideas and paradigms influence the practice of Nepali social workers?
- How does the existing social, cultural, economic, and political context of Nepal influence the work of Nepali social workers?
- What do Nepali social work practitioners say are the key influences on their practice?
- What practices comprise an emerging decolonised and developmental Nepali social work practice approach?
- Are Nepali social workers engaged in decolonising practices, *that is*, how are they tailoring their work to fit local sociostructural issues and problems?
- What might a model of decolonised and developmental social work practice approach look like in the context of Nepal?

Author's positionality and reflexivity in knowledge production

Birks and Mills (2011) noted that positionality assumed a relationship between knowledge production and reflexive practice. The knowledge producer should be a reflexive practitioner. This means being explicit about his or her relationship to the knowledge production and the knowledge keepers and building in measures to equalise power imbalances and increase reciprocity with those who are active actors in knowledge production, *that is*, to the knowledge keepers. To do this, the knowledge producer openly declares his or her assumptions about the phenomenon under study. There was risk that making my assumptions about Nepali social work explicit to the participants would likely have influenced their responses to the exploratory questions and run counter to the bracketing technique grounded theory offered to model decolonised and developmental Nepali social work. Nevertheless, positionality required that I made my epistemological and ontological stance explicit at the outset, since this was fundamental to the qualitative knowledge production process (Crotty, 1998), especially when one embraces decolonial epistemology. I must admit that I am unable to divorce myself from my past experiences and actions that, wittingly or unwittingly, has guided me to this point and has shaped the way I have framed this book, the questions I have asked, the observations and interpretations I have made, and my reporting of the decolonised and developmental Nepali social work. Notwithstanding, I have enhanced the trustworthiness of this book by explicitly locating myself in the narrative, probing my biases throughout, clearly describing my role as an author and my vested interests in the book, as discussed below (Creswell, 2009; Janesick, 2000).

Gilgun and Abrams (2002) suggested that situating the knower in knowledge production was an act exemplifying 'the spirit of reflexivity' (p. 41). Given that 'observations are laden with culture-specific ontologies' (Gordon, 1991, p. 606), I am part of the knowledge production process and the model generated in this book (Charmaz, 2006). Hence, it is essential that I make my position explicit in the book from the very beginning so that readers are not misguided throughout the texts:

- I belong to the same community of Nepali social workers whose world views have contributed to generate the model of decolonised and developmental Nepali social work presented in this book.
- My epistemology and ontology have influenced the knowledge production process.
- I have elicited the conceptual density and thick description required to develop decolonised and developmental social work by establishing a rapport with participants and bracketing my biases.
- My focus has been the meanings social workers attribute to their experience.
- I want to frame decolonised social work practice from the day-to-day experiences of Nepali social workers, expecting they had been influenced by Western theories and models learnt through their education and further embedded by the donor-driven INGOs in which they have been working.
- The model of decolonised and developmental social work I have developed is a collective construction based on my and the knowledge-keepers' shared experience and understanding.
- Others might frame the model of decolonised and developmental Nepali social work in a different way and thus might elicit different world views.
- I have chosen the grounded theory approach because of its synergies with indigenous and decolonising knowledge production and critical pedagogy, as discussed here.

Synergies with indigenous ways of knowing

Indigenous ways of knowing perceive knowledge production as a transformative process in which people's voices must be heard (Hart, 2009; Kovach, 2005, 2009; Smith, 2012). Though my initial ideas about decolonised and developmental Nepali social work had been influenced by critical social work theories, including radical social work (Bailey & Brake, 1975; Lavalette, 2011), Marxist social work (Corrigan, 1978), structural social work (Hick, 2009; Mullaly, 1997, 2002), and post-modern social work (Allan, Briskman, & Pease, 2009; Morley, 2014), none of these theories did justice to my evolving understanding of the indigenisation of social work, defined as 'making Western approaches relevant' (Gray & Hetherington, 2013, p. 25). I saw indigenisation as the left wing of universal social work and the unfinished job of imperialist social work. Given the idea of the indigenisation of social work still draws on Western-informed theories, it could be described as 'brown or black on the outside and white on the inside'. Indigenisation, in other words, has not been 'neutral in its objectification of the Other . . . [and has] clear links to Western knowledge [that has] . . . generated a particular relationship to indigenous peoples which continues to be problematic' (Smith, 2012, p. 39); notwithstanding, many scholars in social work have promoted indigenisation without critical scrutiny.

Indigenous knowledge producers are extremely mindful of the history of white logics and their colonising practices in research and remain suspicious of their epistemological, ontological, and methodological paradigms and their production of fragmented truths and distorted histories (Birks & Mills, 2011; Rigney, 1999; Smith, 2012). What is needed is an approach that deconstructs hegemonic white world views and decolonise knowledge systems embedded by early scholars – Western missionaries, travellers, explorers, and anthropologists, like Hamilton (1819), Hodson (1817), Kirk Patric (1811), and Oldfield (1880) – who had instilled the dominant view of 'cultural romanticism' and 'soul searching' through spirit[ual] possession' (Hitchcock & Jones, 1976 in Devkota, 2007, p. 27) in Nepal. For a time, Nepal became a mecca for Western researchers' personal romanticism and professional development (Devkota, 2007), and in every possible way the knowledge produced in this book seeks to eliminate the similar tradition.

More recently, the space previously occupied by Western missionaries and researchers has been occupied by INGOs, and bilateral and multilateral aid agencies to which many Nepali social workers have been drawn as a source of employment. Nepali social work education and its practice has yet to break down the intellectual colonisation brought by colonial research methodologies and develop its own home-grown research methods to study local peoples' subjective reality. Thus, what is required is an empirical method rooted in Nepali values and norms. To this end, I wonder whether I should develop a completely new methodology or adapt an exisiting methodology. I am mindful of Smith's (2012) observation:

> Decolonization . . . does not mean and has not meant a total rejection of all theory or research or [the] Western knowledge. Rather it is about centering our concerns and worldviews and then coming to know and understand the theory and research from our own perspectives and for our own purpose.
>
> (p. 41)

Also I want to be sure that the methodology that I have chosen for this book does 'not replace the hegemonic order with one that suffocates life and does not allow each of us to flourish in ways that we may not even be able to begin to imagine' (Dei, 2005, p. 12). Transparency and accountability, so central to indigenous or decolonised study, also mean knowledge generated should be communicable to the target peoples, that is, to the Nepali social workers in particular and others with similar expectations in general. Therefore, I discern a pragmatic path to develop the idea of decolonised and developmental Nepali social work in Nepal. A further insight to overcome methodological dilemma came from my PhD supervisor, Professor Mel Gray, who has immensely contributed to the field of indigenous and decolonisation of social work studies (see for instance, Gray et al., 2008a, 2013b). Gray et al. (2013c) had argued that we should no longer use the term 'indigenous social work' within the decolonisation discourse relating to developing countries and wondered whether 'indigenisation' was an outmoded concept and decolonisation more accurately reflected the political project of Indigenous Peoples and the Global South context. Thus, shifting the ground of Western social work in Nepal means detaching it from its existing theoretical perspective and finding a way to study Nepali social work from the ground up.

Smith (1999) highlighted the importance of transparency in indigenous knowledge production; how the knowledge production process is conducted is as important as what is found. 'Processes are expected to be respectful, to enable people, to heal and educate . . . to lead one small step further towards self-determination', Smith (1999, p. 128) argued. Thus, critical questions arise in formulating knowledge production for this book from an indigenist perspective: Whose knowledge is it? Who has designed the question and framed the phenomena of the study? Whose interests will it serve? Who will benefit? Who is writing up this idea? How will the knowledge be disseminated?

Synergising indigenous ways of knowing, the knowledge production for this book has been conducted from a standpoint. It begins with detailed attention to the knower's vested interests, motivation, and positionality (Creswell, 2009). As a Nepali social worker, I am critical of the way in which social work has been imported and embedded into social work education in Nepal, especially since social work is not an officially sanctioned profession and there is no service infrastructure to employ social workers. Therefore, there are no jobs for social work graduates, though some have found employment in INGOs. Thus, the book seeks to gather information about the experiences of Nepali social workers employed in INGOs to develop knowledge on emerging social work practice in Nepal.

Further, social work research has paid scant attention to the 'increased awareness that there are distinct cultural, social, and historical experiences shaping and influencing group experience' (Engel & Schutt, 2013, p. 17). As outlined in Chapter 5, the transfer of social work from the West to the rest suggests a tendency toward cultural stereotyping resulting in an insider/outsider dichotomy (Matsuoka, Morelli, & McCubbin, 2013). Historically, the outsider has silenced and colonised indigenous knowledges, due to the imperialist tendencies of international social work (Midgley, 1981) and its disregard for insider cultural, historical, and contextual knowledge in the process of knowledge production and transfer (Gray & Coates, 2010; Gray et al., 2008b, 2013c; Sinclair, Hart, & Bruyere, 2009).

Given the Nepali population comprised diverse caste and ethnic groups, and diverse languages and dialects, discerning a locally oriented, decolonised practice is a complex undertaking and makes even more difficult by three decades history of Nepali social work relying on its Western roots, as discussed in Chapter 4 and Chapter 5. The methodological challenge is to find an appropriate methodology through which to examine

Nepali social workers' experiences of practice from their insider sociocultural-structural perspective to discern locally relevant practice models of social work. This book, thus, goes beyond description to explore how Nepali social workers interpret and understand their experiences in light of the sociopolitical and cultural environment in which they are constructing practice.

Synergies with a critical theory and thinking

What I had in mind before I started this project was the critical transformation of Western-informed social work to a localised, home-grown model of Nepali social work, through the voices of Nepali social workers as 'voices from the margins [that would reflect] . . . the range of [Nepali] knowledge, perspectives, languages, and ways of being' (Cannella & Lincoln, 2011, p. 83). Such an approach must have synergies with critical pedagogy (Kincheloe, 2007), decolonised methodology (Smith, 2012), Red pedagogy (Grande, 2007), and an ethics of alterity (Ritchie & Rau, 2010). These approaches balance the power between the knower and those being knowledge keepers, positioning them as partners in a collective struggle: 'If you have come to accompany us, if you think our struggle is also your struggle, we have plenty of things to talk about' (Glesne, 2007, p. 171). Critical pedagogy highlights the politics of knowledge production and the colonising tendencies of enlightenment thinking that colonises minds (Butler, 2002; Foucault, 1984). Thus, there is the possibility that Nepali social workers may be uncritical of the social work methods they have been taught in Nepal. How can I, as a knowledge producer, listen openly to their experience, while leading them toward thinking about Nepali social work from a decolonising perspective? From the outset, I understand the interplay of power dynamics between myself (as a knower) and Nepali social workers (as those being knowledge keepers). I have been familiar with Sarantakos's (2005) argument that knowledge is power, hence those who control the knowledge production hold the power. Though I am in control of the knowledge production presented in this book, I am reliant on Nepali social workers' subjective knowledge as a data source, despite their possibly uncritical view (Pelz, 2014; Piety, 2010).

Constructivist grounded theory offers the technique of bracketing, whereby I may contain my assumptions and ideas – my tacit knowledge, belief systems, lived historical experiences, socialisation, culture, socioeconomic status, and educational background – in accessing Nepali social workers' interpretations and experiences from which I model decolonised and developmental social work practice in Nepal latter in this book. Bracketing safeguards me from contaminating Nepali social workers' accounts of practice with my own ideas.

Definition of key terms used in the book

> *Authentisation*, according to Ragab (1982, 2017), refers to the real and critical efforts to recognise all aspects of the social work profession in light of local circumstances and environment.
>
> *Decolonisation* as the process within alternative social work discourse resists the colonising and imperialistic tendencies of Western social work and gives autonomy to local peoples to shape social work according to their social, cultural, and political values.

Indigenisation represents the process of making Western social work fit to non-Western contexts.

Localisation integrates local routinised behaviour in social work knowledge and practice.

'Nepalisation' of social work or Nepali social work refers to Nepali peoples' insider approach and process to transform borrowed Western social work to fit the Nepali context. While doing so, it emphasises Nepal's unique and diverse cultures and the sociostructural issues to which social work seeks to respond.

Way forward

Having introduced the book and its genesis, enquiry method, and purpose in this chapter, Chapter 2 describes the socio-cultural-politico context of the book, beginning with Nepal's complex geography, ecology, and regional dynamics and its unique social, cultural, and political landscape. Chapter 3 examines the INGO sector as the development context employing social workers. Chapter 4 examines social work education in Nepal and, given the paucity of local literature, includes my analysis drawing on personal experiences.

Chapter 5 reviews the literature on decolonising social work and critically analyses interrelated concepts, such as indigenisation, conscientisation, authentisation, localisation, contextualisation, and culturally sensitive social work, and the need for a shift from indigenisation to decolonisation in Nepali social work. Drawing on direct experiences of Nepali social workers, Chapter 6 builds the cases for the decolonised, developmental, and political nature of Nepali social work before presenting the model of decolonised and developmental Nepali social work in Chapter 7. Finally, drawing together the arguments developed across chapters, the book concludes in Chapter 8. It also points out that decolonised and developmental Nepali social work is part of a process rather than a project and therefore scholarships must continue to engage to advance the conceptual meaning of decolonised and developmental Nepali social work in the future.

Chapter 2

The puzzle of Nepali narratives

Historical dynamics and contemporary issues

In this chapter, I discuss the social context of the decolonised and developmental Nepali social work and elucidate the factors affecting social, cultural, and political change in Nepal, political structure, social institutions, and unique lifestyles, and highlight cultural diversity within Asia.

Asia comprises three major regional powers – China, India, and Japan – and several fast-growing economies, often referred as Asian Tigers – Hong Kong, Singapore, South Korea, and Taiwan. Hemmed in by China and India, Westerners know Nepal because of its elegant Himalayas. However, its mountainous terrain, though good for intrepid explorers, has hampered socioeconomic development in poverty-ridden Nepal. Further, a history of conflict and a decade-long Maoist insurgency has devastated the country, leaving it a hotbed of political discontent unable to transition to fully fledged democracy. With 125 ethnic groups, the country has yet to fully implement its controversial Constitution to cater for the diverse interests of its population.

Isolated by its past rulers, Nepal has been an enigma to the outside world. The few who managed to penetrate its borders saw it as a *Shangri-La*, a permanently happy earthly paradise and mythical Himalayan utopia. Since the end of the Rana oligarchy in 1951, Nepal has experimented with an absolute monarchy, *Bahudal,* or multiparty democracy system, Maoist insurgency (modelled on the doctrine of China's Chairman Mao Zedong and Peru's *Shining Path*), and federal republic, all in the name of freedom, development, and democracy. However, Nepali society remains hampered by stagnant economic growth, locked in political transition and failed social transformation.

Geography, ecology, and regional dynamics

Tucked in the foothills of the Himalaya Mountains, between China to the north and India to the west, south, and east, Nepal is a small, landlocked country with a population of about 28.9 million people (World Bank, 2018). Sill and Kirkby (2013) described it as a gigantic natural stairway from the low-lying Terai to the soaring Himalayas, before taking a deep dive towards the Tibetan Plateau. In its about 100-mile span from north to south, Nepal's altitude ranges from a few 100 feet to the highest mountain peak in the world, Mount Everest. Its climate varies from sub-zero temperatures in the Himalayas to over 100 degrees Fahrenheit in the sub-tropical humid lowland of the Terai.

Administratively, Nepal comprises seven provinces (see Figure 2.1), 77 districts, 293 municipalities including metropolitan and sub-metropolitan cities, and 460 rural municipalities as follows:

1   The Province One comprises 14 districts, 49 municipalities, and 88 rural municipalities.
2   The Province Two comprises eight districts, 77 municipalities, and 59 rural municipalities.
3   The Province Three comprises 13 districts, 45 municipalities, and 74 rural municipalities.
4   The Province Four comprises 11 districts, 27 municipalities, and 58 rural municipalities.
5   The Province Five comprises 12 districts, 36 municipalities, and 73 rural municipalities.
6   The Province Six comprises ten districts, 25 municipalities, and 54 rural municipalities.
7   The Province Seven comprises nine districts, 34 municipalities, and 54 rural municipalities.

(Government of Nepal [GoN], 2017)

Nepal has three physiographic regions: (i) Himalaya; (ii) mountain; and (iii) Terai (see Figure 2.2). Situated at 12,000 feet above sea level, the Himalayas occupy 15 percent of Nepal's total land area. The harsh snow-covered topography makes life arduous for the 6.73 percent of the population living in the Himalayan region. This largely nomadic pastoral population move with their livestock between the Himalayan highlands in the summer and the low-lying valleys in the winter. Long a means of livelihoods, trade with Tibet came to a halt with its annexation by China in the late 1950s.

Nepal's Himalayan range has two major ecological functions. First, it forms a natural wall that blocks freezing arctic air from entering inner Asia. Second, it is a major hydraulic force in that the moist clouds from the Bay of Bengal collide with the mountains to form monsoons that determine the fate of thousands of farmers in the country, and it is the source of rivers that provide spring water, irrigation, and hydropower to many of Nepali populations (Shrestha, 2002).

Nepal's large mountainous region varies between latitudes of approximately 900 and 8000 feet and is home to 43 percent of Nepal's population. The mountains are categorised into high mountains (6000–82000 feet), middle mountains (2000–6000 feet), and lower mountains (900–2000 feet). The mountain inhabitants have dominated people's sociocultural and political lives since the inception of the Nepali state. However, like the Himalayas, its geographical complexities obstruct development in the mountains resulting in poor accessibility to transport, education, and health services. Further, natural calamities, such as landslides, erosion, and floods, compound the misery of Nepal's mountain people, especially during the monsoon season.

The topography, climate, and social lives of people in the Terai are completely different from those in the other two regions. Straddling the Gangetic plain of India, the Terai flatland, where half (50.27 percent) of Nepal's population lives, comprises only 17 percent of the country's landmass. Until the 1950s, the Terai was a malaria hub that, through natural biological warfare, protected Nepal from the British East India Company, which had colonised India. Also, Nepal's aristocrats and upper social classes – its dominant political leaders – laid claim to the bountiful Terai. To this day, the Terai constitutes a vote bank for Nepal's political leaders. Relative to the other two regions, most of its inhabitants are economically deprived and socially and politically marginalised (Shrestha, 2002).

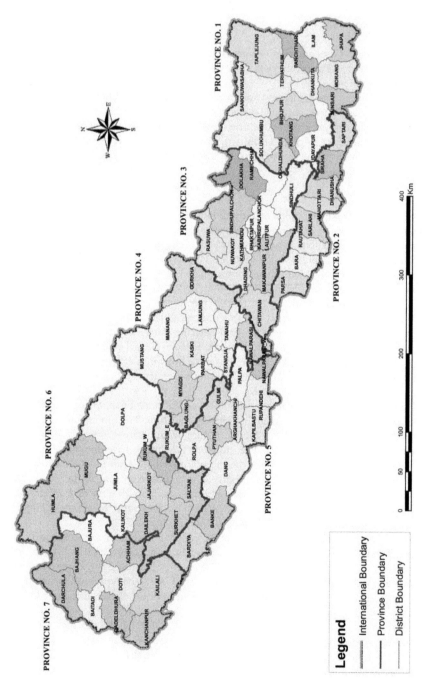

Figure 2.1 Provinces of Nepal

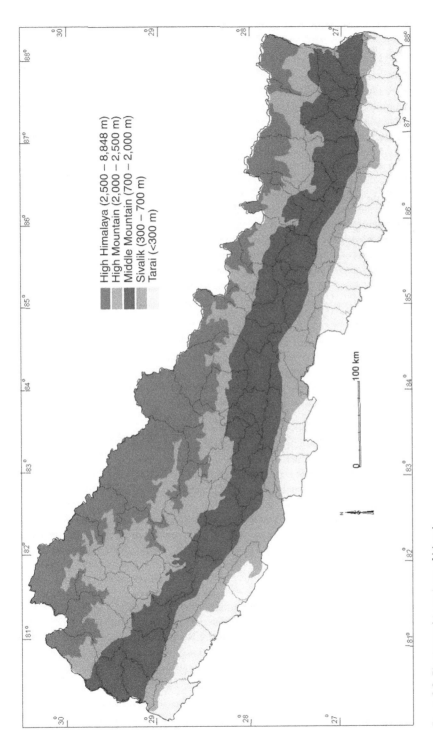

High Himalaya (2,500 – 8,848 m)
High Mountain (2,000 – 2,500 m)
Middle Mountain (700 – 2,000 m)
Sivalik (300 – 700 m)
Tarai (<300 m)

100 km

Figure 2.2 Physiographic regions of Nepal

From a yam between two boulders to a gradual shift to the north

Opinions on Nepal's geostrategic position vary from conformist to historical revisionist. Conformists view Nepal as a yam (an elongated vegetable similar in shape to its landmass) between two boulders (India and China), as poetically described by King Prithvi Narayan Shah in the late 18th century. He believed the country's future hinged on harmonious relations with China and India (Ishii & Karan, 1997). By contrast, many young Nepalis are historical revisionists, who see Nepal as a needle between two balloons (Ghimire, 2015), a hotbed of conspiracy, trading political ideologies devised by think tanks in Beijing and Delhi that could burst at any point.

Chaturvedi and Malone (2012) believed Nepal's internal and external policies had always pivoted around three main objectives: maintaining internal stability, pursuing independent national policies, and gaining a footing in regional and international relations. From the outset, this has remained a critical factor for Nepali policymakers. As Rose (1969) highlighted in the second half of the 20th century, Nepali people 'tend to view their homeland as an intermediate zone between South and Central Asia, belonging to both regions but . . . exclusively affiliated with [neither]' (p. 357). Given Nepal's fragile political and economic situation, and its acquiescence to Beijing and New Delhi, none of these goals were realistically attainable. Consequently, the bilateral stranglehold of Beijing and New Delhi dwarfed national interests.

Chaturvedi and Malone (2012) described Nepal's relations with India as a joyless psychodrama in which neither side could be satisfied. The sociocultural and geographical links and open borders between Nepal and India conjured up a brief relationship of bond and bile. Nepal's attempts to become an equal neighbour rested on the inversion of the unequal Treaty of Peace and Friendship signed with India in 1950; India continued its coercive diplomacy and big brother attitude to which Nepal felt 'a mix of dependence, victimization, solicitude, awe, and resentment' (Chaturvedi & Malone, 2012, p. 298). India's interests in Nepal were, *inter alia*, its resistance to China's growing influence and Pakistani-affiliated madrassa, its desire to protect its open border with Nepal, and to gain control over its abundant hydropower. China's twin concerns complicated India's relationship with Nepal as that growing superpower exerted a gradual influence over South Asia through Nepal. Moreover, China feared that Nepal might foster Nepali-Tibetan anti-China sentiments (Mathou, 2005).

Regarding overseas influences, there was speculation that, as in Afghanistan and Iraq, the USA would continue to engage in Nepal as a non-geostrategic power (Chaturvedi & Malone, 2012). Initially, during the Maoist insurgency, Washington's approach was not only to defend the monarchy by providing aid, equipment, and training to the royal armies fighting the Maoist guerrillas, but also to halt any *entente cordiale* between Nepal's political parties and the Maoists. Hence, its allegiance shifted. Though Washington's battle was for freedom and democracy around the world, many in Nepali civil society found the USA's intervention part of the problem rather than the solution to the country's political transition (Jha, 2012). Though the Maoists became the biggest political party and formed a government after the first constitutional assembly election in 2007, the US State Department continued to enlist them as terrorist until 2012 (Taylor, 2012). Thus, Nepal was trapped inside a triangle of regional – China and India – and non-regional – the USA – powers.

Critical junctures in the making of the Nepali state

Prior to the establishment of the Shah Dynasty, Gopal, Mahispal, Lichhavi, and Malla dynasties ruled the capital, Kathmandu. The Gopal and Lichhavi dynasties initiated the nation state and established the Pashupati Temple (one of the biggest symbols of Hinduism in Nepal), while extending international relationships and religious development, and managing settlement areas for local peoples (Chalise, 1992; Dahal, 1992). History recognised the prehistoric Lichhavi period as a 'Golden Era', due to the rulers' efforts to integrate peoples' participation in state structures, organise human life, provide standard economic provision, uplift educational levels, and develop the arts (Chalise, 1992). The Medieval Period, dominated by the Mallas dynasty, witnessed immense social and economic reforms to develop Nepal's physical infrastructure, institute social welfare programs, improve business and commerce, provide land for homeless and poor people, and introduce capital punishment (Chalise, 1992; Dahal, 1992):

> Community work or [the] concept of social organization was developed in the form of *guthi* [and] *Raj guthi* [clan or caste-based informal organisation], *and sewa khalak* [clan or caste-based service organisation] for the welfare of family, group and community. Importantly, *guthi, Raj guthi and sewa khalak* had played [a] significant role in cultural and religious development along with community development and maintaining family and social order.
>
> (Shrestha, 2013, p. 15)

The Shah dynasty laid the foundations of the modern Nepal as it progressed through the Shah (1768–1846), Rana (1846–1951), brief transition (1951–1962), and *Panchayat* system – a partyless, monarchical system (1962–1990) – periods to the most recent period of democratic transition and disillusionment from 1990 onwards. Modern-day Nepal came into existence in the mid-18th century when King Prithvi Narayan Shah of Gorkha, then a tiny kingdom, launched his military expansion. He commanded an army comprised mostly of *Janajatis* (a Nepali word for Indigenous Peoples), such as the *Magar* and *Gurung*, led by upper warrior caste Kshatriya. Possibly one of the strategic rulers, equipped with logistical acumen and political skills, Prithvi Narayan Shah combined conciliation and intimidation in equal measure, not only to conquer small kingdoms but also to expand his territories over the fringes of modern-day India's east, north, and northwest. From his accession in 1743, he fought the peoples of the Kathmandu Valley, finally capturing this region in 1768. By the time of his death in 1775, he had occupied most of eastern Nepal and modern Sikkim in India (Whelpton, 2005).

Despite the formal end of the monarchy in 2008, Prithvi Narayan Shah, the founder of the modern-day Nepal, remained a celebrated hero, portrayed in Nepali history, literature, and academic texts as one of the greatest nationalists ever born in the land of Nepal. However, post-colonial and anti-hegemonic discourses questioned his imperialist unification of Nepal and labelled his military conquest as the dawn of dispossession, ethnocide, and forced acculturation for millions of ethnics and *Janajatis* on the margins of Nepali society (von Einsiedel, Malone, & Pradhan, 2012b; Pradhan, 1991; Whelpton, 2005). Rather than unify Nepal, von Einsiedel, Malone, and Pradhan (2012a) argued that the Shah's invasion of the Indo-Aryan Terai and Tibeto-Burman hill people's territories eroded their unique cultures and lifestyles and undermined their traditional governance structures. To this day, Nepal's *Janajatis* and ethnic minorities struggle to survive imperialistic and modernising forces:

> Before unification, tribal, ethnic, linguistic, and social caste groups in Nepal's constituent parts pursued their affairs largely autonomously within their own small borders. The Nepali state's expansion forced these myriad groups to live together under the authority of the new Gorkha rulers. By the time Nepal's [coercive] unification was completed, Nepali society had become multicultural, multiethnic, and multilingual. The failure to recognize and accommodate [them] through active nurturing this new reality . . . [has continued] to trouble Nepal in the ensuing centuries'.
>
> (von Einsiedel et al., 2012a, p. 5)

Pradhan (1991) argued that Prithvi Narayan Shah's state making through warfare created a tenuous unity, at best. Like Henry V of England, he emerged as a barbaric emperor from the small hill kingdom of Gorkha threatening his neighbouring rulers. He acted ruthlessly, after conquering Kirtipur – a small town situated to the southwest of Kathmandu – and ordering his armies to cut off the lips and noses of the inhabitants. Today such actions would constitute war crimes and gross human rights violations (Vaidya, 1993).

The Shah dynasty's voracious territorial expansion ended when the British East India Company defeated Nepali armies in 1816. Consequently, Nepal signed the *Sugauli Treaty* ceding all conquered territories in India to the British. Since then Nepal has not been able to add even an inch of land through military invasion. The British East India Company returned some parts of its western districts in exchange for Nepali support in suppressing the Indian Sepoy Mutiny in 1857 (von Einsiedel et al., 2012a).

Importantly, between 1768 and 1846, the royal family, including the ministers, aides, and officials inside the court, were more concerned about centralising power than state building or human development. Janga Bahadur Rana, an ambitious military leader serving at the court, saw divisions in the royal family and their aides as an opportunity to seize power. In 1846, he instituted his autocratic Rana regime through an internally initiated colonisation process and a bloody coup, popularly known as *Kot Parva*. The Rana regime ruled Nepal for the next 104 years. Rana's nepotistic rulers kept a powerless monarchy in place, while isolating Nepal from the outside, preventing Westerners from entering the country, in as far as was possible, and allowing conditional access to education for Nepali citizens. In 1854, they promulgated the *Muluki Ain*, that is, civil code dividing the population into a caste structure and hierarchy that resulted in large-scale sanctioned discrimination and marginalisation (see Table 2.1). Horizontal caste discrimination practices were deeply rooted in Nepali society, restricting access to resources for those with low social status (Whelpton, 2005).

Despite their autocratic system of governance, some Rana prime ministers contributed to progress and development. For example, the fourth Rana Prime Minister, Dev Shamsher, established vernacular schools, abolished female slavery in the Kathmandu valley, and introduced Nepal's first newspaper, the *Gorkhapatra*. Thereafter, Chandra Shamsher abolished *Sati* (a Hindu practice, whereby widows burn to death on their husband's funeral pyre) and slavery in Nepal. His most visible legacy is the Trichandra College, Nepal's first, and Singh Durbar, which houses most of the government secretariats today.

The execution of four martyrs in 1941 marked growing dissatisfaction with the Rana regime. The newly founded NCP (formed in India in 1947) and the politically

Table 2.1 Nepali social hierarchy in 1854

Hierarchy	Habitat	Religion
A) Water acceptable (Pure) – *Pani Chalne Jat*		
1. Wearers of the sacred thread *(Tagadhari)*		
'Upper caste' Brahmans and Chhetris	Hills	Hinduism
(Parbatiya – hill Hindus)	Terai	Hinduism
'Upper caste' (Madhesi)	Kathmandu	Hinduism
'Upper caste' (Newar)	Valley	
2. Matwali alcohol drinkers (non-enslavable)		
Gurung, Magar, Sunuwar, Thakali, Rai,	Hills	Tribal/Shamanism
Limbu Newar	Kathmandu Valley	Buddhism
3. Matawali alcohol drinkers (enslavable)		
Bhote (including Tamang)	Mountains/Hills	Buddhism
Chepang, Gharti, Hayu	Hills	Animism
Kumal, Tharu	Inner Terai	
B) Water un-acceptable (Impure) – *Pani Nachalne Jat*		
4. Touchable		
Dhobi, Kasai, Kusale, Kulu	Kathmandu Valley	Hinduism
Musalman [or Muslim]	Terai	Islam
Mlechha (foreigner)	Europe	Christianity, etc.
5. Untouchable (achut)		
Badi, Damai, Gaine, Kadara, Kami, Sarki	Hills	Hinduism
(Parbatiya – hill Hindus)	Kathmandu	Hinduism
Chyame, Pode (Newar)	Valley	

Source: Adapted from Gurung (2002, in Bennett, Dilli, & Govindasamy, 2008, p. 2)

impotent King Tribhuvan later led an anti-Rana movement. Nepal's suppressed peoples and Prime Minister Nehru in India, newly independent from the grip of the British East India Company, also supported anti-Rana initiatives. India facilitated political consensus between the king, NCP, and the Ranas, which formally ended the Rana regime and ushered in the first democracy in 1951.

Between 1951 and 1960, there was a sudden rise in the number of political parties from all ideological persuasions, including the communist party, founded in India in 1949. Rather than strengthening the infant democracy, King Tribuvan began to claw back power, not only from the still-entrenched Rana clans, but also from Nepal's nascent political parties. Until he died, King Tribhuvan kept himself busy by routinely changing prime ministers, while the promised constitutional assembly never materialised. Thus, King Tribhuvan reinvigorated an autocratic monarchy that blossomed under his successor King Mahendra and ended when King Birendra, 11th heir of the Shah dynasty, restored democracy in 1990. King Mahendra's legacies are controversial and the jury is out on whether he was an autocratic architect of development or an extreme nationalist, who turned Nepal's cultural mosaic into a boiling melting pot. In 1960, King Mahendra instituted the *Panchayat* system and dissolved the parliament formed after the first general election in 1959. With strong backing from the royal armies, he succeeded in pushing Nepal's political parties to the edge. Despite his infrastructure-building development programs, his regime bred corruption, nepotism, and favouritism that have proved extremely difficult to eradicate in contemporary Nepal.

Nepali students in government universities and colleges, always more active in politics than the common citizen, protested against the *Panchayat* system in 1979. The ruling monarch, King Birendra, called for a referendum, which voted in favour of keeping the *Panchayat* system in place (Whelpton, 2005). Subsequent world events in the 1980s, such as *Perestroika* in Russia and the fall of the Berlin Wall in Germany, reinvigorated the youth movement's call for democracy. Youth agitation turned to a nationwide revolt, popularly known as the *Jana Aandolan I* (or People's Movement I), in which the underground political parties, professional classes, trade unions, and citizen groups called for the restoration of democracy. The many political parties based in India and the Indian government forced King Birendra to restore a multiparty democratic system in 1990 (Whelpton, 2005). However, the ensuing political transition failed to produce improvements in socioeconomic well-being (Pfaff-Czarnecka, 2004a, 2004b). Rural disparities, bonded labour, untouchability, women's oppression, unequal access to education and health, and ethnic-based discrimination continued in the face of the poor performance of state politicians and administrators. This stagnation led to growing disillusionment among the people and the advent of the Maoist insurgency in the western hills of Nepal in 1996, which led to the death of hundreds and thousands of people.

At the beginning of 20th century, the last monarch, King Gyanendra, declared a state of emergency following the royal massacre and brutal Maoist attacks on the police and army in the hills. The major political parties formed the Seven Parties Alliance (SPA) comprising the NCP, NCP-Democratic, Communist Party Nepal – United Marxist Leninist, Sadbhavana (Anandi Devi), Jana Morcha Nepal, Samyukta Baam Morcha, and Nepal Workers and Peasants parties. They signed a 12-point Memorandum of Understanding with Maoists, under the Indian government's mediation, as the SPA formed the *Jana Aandolan II* (or People's Movement II) between 2006 and 2007. After its success in ending the 240-year monarchy, the SPA led an interim government and peacebuilding process. Thus, Nepal departed from a Hindu-dominated monarchic system to a secular Federal Democratic Republic with an interim constitution, government, and constitution assembly. The SPA promised for a 'New Nepal', with inclusive, democratic, and progressive governance to end the autocratic centralised system that had long dominated the Nepali political landscape.

In January 2007, the *Madhesh* Movement (also known as *Madhesh Aandolan*) in the flatlands of eastern and central part of the Terai, among peoples who shared a common culture and dialects with the people of north India, demanded recognition and inclusion in the state apparatus. *Madheshi* issues reached the attention of national politicians and international development actors and rights defenders. In the wake of the *Madhesh* Movement, dozens of armed groups and secessionist emerged in the Terai, actively threatening the Nepali government to the present day.

Following two constituent assemblies, several strikes, countless pennies, six prime ministers, and eight years in office, Nepal finally delivered the Constitution of Nepal in October 2015, despite complaints from the marginalised *Dalits*, indigenous (or

Janajatis), Madheshis, and Muslims (also known as DIMM), and women's organisations. However, there is no quick fix to Nepal's complex development woes. Thus, to date, it remains a failed nation state (Rotberg, 2003).

Revisiting Nepali history: one step forward, two steps back

The history of Nepal is more than a mere recording of events. It comprises cultural narratives that have shaped Nepali society and its diverse peoples. The political history outlined above provided three major insights about Nepal – the making of the patrimonial state, the institutionalisation of hegemonic ideologies, and a litany of failed development (Panday, 1999, 2012). Nepal's state apparatus comprises political leaders, public officials, bureaucrats, and soldiers tasked with implementing social policy and ensuring the nation's physical security through its established institutions. Its economic and political power extends beyond the public to the private domain, and legislation and the machinations of government legitimised its authority. The state is responsible for Nepal's transformation from a pre-capitalist and pre-industrialist society to a dynamic and progressive nation (Khan, 2002). Drawing on European experiences, Tilly (1975, 1985) proposed that state formation proceeded through four phases:

1   War or territorial advancement by force.
2   Elimination or neutralisation of potential threats within the territory.
3   Protection for supporters to sustain new structures of governance.
4   Extraction of resources through taxation.

These phases loosely conform to the making of the Nepali state. The ruling elites and high castes often dominated its history, which Riaz and Basu (2010) described as a 'roving banditry', using taxes for their personal gain rather than to foster socio-economic development. Feudalistic and patrimonial practices to control *Janajatis* and ethnic populations propagated this banditry. One such practice was *Birta* – a strategy of the ruling elites to appease the upper castes through land grants that placed agricultural land, which sustained the peasantry, under the control of feudal landlords (Regmi, 1976; Riaz & Basu, 2010). This system typified the elitist colonising practices that undermined the cultural and linguistic autonomy of Nepal's *Janajatis* and ethnic peoples and denied them their democratic rights. As Lawoti (2003) explained,

> Hill caste Hindu elite males . . . [dominated] politics, administrations, the judiciary, parliament, academia, civil society, industry/commerce, local government, and education . . . [all] important arenas of governance . . . the political leaders, especially the top leadership, can exercise unrestrained power, appointing sycophants to administrative posts, ignoring party rules and procedures, and often governing on their personal whims. The leaders nominate at least half of the central committee members, often relatives (such as the [NCP]), and/or caste brethren (as in the [Communist Party Nepal-United Marxist Leninist]). The appointees in turn, remain personally loyal to the leaders. Leaders also appoint party candidates for parliamentary, local, and organization elections.
>
> (p. 52)

This strange brew of roving banditry, feudalism, and patrimony inevitably led to under-development and gross inequalities in Nepal like the conditions in Nigeria described by Kimuyu (1999):

> [When the] government behaves like roving bandits, they are unlikely to have a development agenda that can be shared with those that they seek to govern. Improvement in the citizen's [sic] quality of life would therefore be accidental. Under the roving bandit form of government, the evolution of development poli-cies is also unlikely, considering the absence of clear goals future. Such forms of government cannot encourage the evolution of clear rules and enforcement mechanisms through which private interests for the benefit of the community can be encouraged. On the contrary, self-seeking governments tend to stifle the devel-opmental outcomes of atomistic behaviour [sic]. Such governments also encourage the birth of parallel systems of micro-governance that find expression in parallel activities, which undermine broader development efforts.
>
> (n.p.)

How did the ruling elite maintain its grip on the Nepali citizenry for so long? The answer lies in the layers of Hindu myths formed around the king, national heroes, and selective nationalism. The king was seen as a descendent of the Hindu god, Vishnu, and protector of the kingdom. The Hindunisation of *Janajatis* nationalities and ethnic identities became a national charter, for not only national unity, but also social status, when the Rana regime introduced *Muluki Ain* to embed the caste system. As a result, a large number of the *Janajatis* and ethnic population became untouchable and so denied citizenship – political and social – rights. The dominant hill culture and language propagated Nepali national-ism. The nationalising *Panchayat* system, introduced by King Mahendra, aimed at Nepal's *Janajatis* and ethnic populations, with their diverse cultures and languages, attempted to make Nepal a melting pot with its rhetoric of *ek bhasa, ek bhesh, ek desh* (one language, one form of dress, one country). This limited vision of nationalism not only slowed develop-ment but also bred conflict and the Maoist insurgency. Despite a brief spell of pluralism and secularism, this nationalistic call for a single language (Nepali), dress (*Daura Suruwal* and *Topi*), and religion (Hinduism) was rekindled in 2007 (von Einsiedel et al., 2012a). This conspiratorial, culturally homogenising hegemony is difficult to challenge in Nepal, since caste elites and intellectual leaders have institutionalised it as a symbol of political solidarity. Today, Nepal's dominant elite rules by 'consent rather than domination, integration rather than exclusion, and co-optation rather than suppression' (Riaz & Basu, 2010, p. 12). The reactionary political movements, most notably the Maoist insurgency, have been unable to release the masses from the long-established structures of Hinduism, casteism, and con-spiracy. Hence, Rotberg (2003) references the failed state. Without social and political transformation, Riaz and Basu (2010) predict a future of violence:

> In the form of civil war directed against the state; the predatory and oppressive nature [of] the state resulting in persecution of its own citizens; inability of the state to control its own territory; growth of the criminal violence and lawlessness posing a threat to the security of the people; deterioration and/or destruction of physical infrastructure; the decaying state of social services (including education and health); and . . . economic opportunity for a few at the expense of the major-ity of the population.
>
> (p. 19)

Sociocultural groups of Nepal: cleavage, conflict, and new politics

The presence of 125 caste and ethnic groups, 123 spoken languages, and ten religions make Nepal a multiethnic, multilinguistic, and multireligious nation. Nepal's last census in 2011 reported that Hinduism (81.3 percent) was the dominant religion, followed by Buddhism (9 percent), Islam (4.4 percent), Kirat – animism and shamanism practised by *Janajatis* and ethnic groups of the Himalayas (3.1 percent) – and Christianity (1.4 percent). Despite its religious and ethnic diversity, Hinduism and the caste system dominate Nepal's sociocultural and political relations (GoN, 2012b). Lawoti (2012) listed *Madheshis*, Caste Hill Hindu Elite (CHHE), *Janajatis*/ethnic, and *Dalits* as the major caste/ethnic categories in terms of political influence and dominance in Nepal (see Table 2.2).

- *Madhesis*: They are inhabitants of the southern plain region with similar languages, cultures, and lifestyles who often use north Indian dialects. The major caste groups in the Terai are Twice-born – Brahmins (0.50 percent), Rajputs (0.15 percent), Kayastha (0.16 percent); pure castes – Yadav (3.97 percent), Kumahars (2.34 percent), Kushwahas (1.17 percent), Kurmis (0.87 percent), Mallahs (0.65 percent), Kewats (0.58 percent), and Halwais (0.31 percent); and Impure castes – Telis (1.39 percent), Kalwars (0.48 percent), and Dhobis (0.41 percent). *Madheshis* also includes 4.4 percent of Muslims (GoN, 2012b).
- *CHHE*: The CHHE includes Brahmin, Kshtriya, Thakuri, and Dashnamis who share same language (Nepali), religion (Hinduism), and lifestyle, including dress. Although it comprises less than a third of the population (31.05 percent) (GoN, 2012b), it dominates Nepal's sociopolitical and cultural landscape (Singh & Kukreja, 2014).
- *Janajatis/ethnics*: *Janajatis* nationalities are native groups with traditional homeland in both hill and Terai. The *Janajatis* people, with a traditional homeland and unique culture, make up around 36 percent of the population in the country. The 2011 census reported that 63 *Janajatis* groups were scattered throughout the Himalayas, the mountains, and the Terai of Nepal. Among these, their access to the state's resources privileges Newar, who constitute 4.98 percent of the total population of the country (GoN, 2012b). However, Lawoti (2012) noted that the state's effort is negligent to support the promotion of Newar's culture and language. Tamangs (4.98 percent), Magars (7.12 percent), Rais (2.34 percent), Sherpas (0.42 percent), and Chepang (0.25 percent) are some major hill origin *Janajatis* population largely speaking the Tibeto-Burman language. The brave Gurkha or Gorkha armies, as the world popularly knows, are mostly from Tamang, Magars, and Rais ethnic groups. Tharus (6.55 percent) are the largest *Madheshi Janajatis* groups followed by Dhanuks (0.82 percent), Rajbanshis (0.43 percent), Kumals (0.47 percent), Majhis (0.31 percent), Danuwars (0.31 percent), Gangais (0.13 percent), Dhimals (0.09 percent), and Darais (0.06 percent) living in *Terai* or *Madhesh* (GoN, 2012b). Unlike hill *Janajatis*, many of the *Madheshis Janajatis* groups share a similar language, culture, and tradition of north India. These ethnic groups are scattered throughout the low belt of Nepal from east to west.
- *Dalit*: They belong to the lowest position in the caste hierarchy and are considered untouchable. They are also considered impure which denies their social and cultural mobility at private and public spaces. They constitute 13.52 percent of the total population. Further, the *Dalits*, speaking both the dominant language Nepali

Table 2.2 Some major caste and ethnic groups of Nepal

Speaking north Indian dialect including Awadhi, Maithali, and Bhojpuri			Hill origin Nepali-speaking		
Twice-born	Brahmins	0.5%	Twice-born	Brahmins	12.17%
	Rajputs	0.15%		Kshetris	16.5%
	Kayasthas	0.16%		Thakuris	1.60%
Pure castes	Yadavs (herdsmen)	3.97%	Renouncers	Dashnamis	0.85%
	Kushawahas (vegetable growers)	1.17%			
	Kurmis (cultivators)	0.87%			
	Mallahs (fishermen)	0.65%			
	Kewats (fishermen)	0.58%			
	Kumahars (porters)	2.34%			
	Halwais (confectioners)	0.31%			
Impure castes	Kalwars (brewers)	0.48%			
	Dhobis (washermen)	0.41%			
	Telis (oilpressers)	1.39%			
Muslims		4.4%			

| | Madheshi | CHHE | |
	Dalit	Janajatis/ethnic	Newar, Tibeto-Burman, Nepali-speaking
Hill origin Nepali-speaking			
Untouchables			Newar 4.98%
Kamis (metal workers) 4.57%			Magars 7.12%
Damais (tailors) 1.78%			Tamangs 5.81%
Sarkis (cobblers) 1.41%			Rais 2.34%
			Gurungs 1.97%
Madheshis			Limbus 1.46%
Untouchables			Sherpas 0.42%
Chamars (leather workers) 1.26%			Chepangs 0.25%
Dushadhs (basket makers) 0.78%			Sunuwars 0.21%
Khatwes (labourers) 0.38%			Bhotiyas 0.05%
Mushhars (labourers) 0.88%			Thakalis 0.04%
			Thamis 0.1%
			Madheshis
			Kumals 0.47%
			Majhis 0.31%
			Danuwars 0.31%
			Darais 0.06%
			Tharus 6.55%
			Dhanuks 0.82%
			Rajbanshis 0.43%
			Gangais 0.13%

Source: Adapted from GoN (2012b). Others (n = 80) have a smaller population than those mentioned in Table 2.2

and north Indian dialect, such as Awadhi, Maithali, and Bhojpuri, are inhabitants of both hill and Terai. The hill *Dalits*, such as Kamis (4.57 percent), Damais (1.78 percent), and Sarkis (1.41 percent) have comparatively better social and political status than some of the *Madheshis Dalits* such as Chamars (1.26 percent), Dushads (0.78 percent), and Khatwes (0.38 percent) (GoN, 2012b). Worth noting, those who fall in more than one subgroup face double discrimination, as it has been seen in the case of *Madheshi Dalit*.

As in India, the caste system remains the dominant social structure in Nepal. It is based on a Hindu classification of hereditary groups (*varnas*) that determines vertical (hierarchical) and horizontal relations (Sharma, 1997). Over its 2000-year history, it has developed into a complex system irreducible to class that combines many elements from birthright and ethnicity to occupation, power, and financial acumen. However, when this caste system encounters the class structure, high caste groups limit the status of lower caste groups by controlling the labour market and segregating jobs and social roles, for instance, as was seen in the disproportionate representation of *Madheshis, Janajatis,* and *Dalit vis-à-vis* CHHE in bureaucratic roles (see Figure 2.3). It has given rise to a discriminatory, oppressive social system, which exploits and marginalises the power-less lower castes (Gellner, 2010; Gurung, 2005, 2006; Jones & Boyd, 2011; Murshed & Gates, 2005; Rao, 2010; Young, 2009).

Although the representation of *Madheshis* has increased in 2009 (8.93 percent) from 2005 (3.03 percent) and 1999 (7.69 percent), it is still lower than their representation

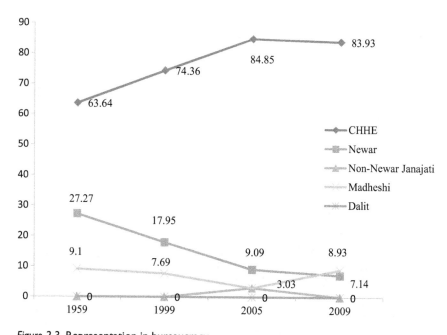

Figure 2.3 Representation in bureaucracy

Source: Adapted from Lawoti (2012), Neupane (2005), and United Nations Development Program (UNDP) (2009)

in 1959 (9.1 percent). Even Newar's representation has constantly dropped from 27.27 percent in 1959 to 17.95 percent in 1999, 9.09 percent in 2005, and 7.14 percent in 2009. There are zero percent representations of non-Newar *Janajatis* and *Dalit* in bureaucratic roles in 2009. The poor representation of *Dalit* and *Madheshis* represents injustice that is the result of higher caste and ethnic control over socioeconomic resources, explained by Mittra and Kumar (2004):

> Caste discrimination is deeply ingrained in Nepali society and widely practiced, especially in rural areas . . . [lower castes] have no advocates within the Nepali high-caste establishment . . . [which lead low castes to] suffer discrimination in innumerable ways, notable in terms of access to education, health care . . . [and] jobs.
>
> (p. 93)

Until the country's leadership collectively accommodates diversified caste and ethnic groups within mainstream sociopolitical structures, terms like secular, federal, democratic, and republic remain hollow. Hence the 'reorganization of [social, economic, and political] institutions and practice of decision making, altering of the division of labor, and similar measures of institutional, structural, and cultural change' (Young, 2009, p. 63) must be a priority. For this, Nepal needs to train social agents, including social workers, and instil knowledge about Nepal's social, cultural, and political history and the disproportionate representation of *Janajatis, Dalit,* and *Madheshi,* in the constituent assemblies of 2008 (see Figure 2.4) and 2013.

Janajatis, Madheshi, and *Dalit,* relative to their distribution in the total population, 36 percent, 32.2 percent, and 13.5 percent, had only 35.61 percent, 24.1 percent, and 8.15 percent representation, respectively, in the Constituent Assembly formed in 2008. In the subsequent Constituent Assembly of 2013, which promulgated the constitution in 2015, CHHE comprised 55.4 percent followed by 22.1 percent *Janajatis,* 15.4 percent *Madheshi,* and 0.4 percent hill *Dalit* in the first-past-the-post electoral system result (UN Nepal, 2013). Lawoti (2012) speculated this could be the result of the lack of inclusive state building, but CHHE has no interest in democratising

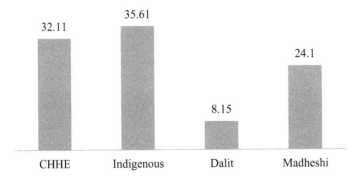

Figure 2.4 Representation in the Constituent Assembly of 2008

Source: Adapted from Lawoti (2012)

the political system. Since the formation of the Nepalit state, all the executive heads (prime ministers) have come from CHHE, with the exception of the first *Madheshi* titular head of state (president, 2007–2015) who had limited power and mainly performed ceremonial functions.

Cultural imperialism and violence persist as marginalised populations find themselves 'defined from the outside . . . [by] those with whom they do not identify and who do not identify with them' (Young, 2009, p. 66). However, DIMM movements are challenging CHHE's dominance and the inclusion of marginalised groups in the state's decision-making structures is improving piecemeal (Lawoti, 2012).

Quest for inclusion, rights, and justice: revisiting the people's movements and Maoist insurgency

Nepal's 1990 'unarmed insurrection' (Schock, 2005; Zunes, 1994) was an organised challenge by people to oppose the *Panchayat* system, demanding freedom of expression, the right to political association and social justice, including the right to form political parties and their sister organisations. The second challenge in 2006, supported by Maoist rebels, led to the abolition of the monarchy. These events leading to the two people's movements, discussed above, are summarised in Table 2.3.

In terms of Brinton's (1965) anatomy of revolution, the 1990 movement resulted from a backlash against the *Panchayat* system, the declining economic situation, widespread political instability, and stagnant development. Collectively these factors left most of the Nepali people with limited freedom and constrained development. Broadbased participation on various political fronts, including the NCP and United Leftist Front, coalesced into a National People's Movement, which delivered a multiparty democracy.

However, in the post-1990 'convalescence' (Brinton, 1965), a period of fragile politics with short-lived governments ensued. There followed the beginning of the Maoist insurgency in 1996 and King Gyanendra's royal takeover dissolving the House of Representatives in 2002, which adversely affected his rule. As in the movement of 1990, Nepali people played a crucial role by agitating for change, defying curfews, holding sit-in strikes, and occupying the streets. The Maoist insurgency was a turning point for the quest for rights, justice, and inclusion. Inspired by Mao Zedong's radical doctrine 'power comes from barrel of the gun' and Peru's 'Shining Path', its adherents believed freedom for Nepal's mainly rural, economically deprived low caste and *Janajatis* was only possible through violent class struggle. However, as with all Nepal's political parties, the CHHE continues to dominate the Maoist party leadership. Moreover, Nepali Maoists were the advance guard of a second-wave world revolution; by establishing their base in Nepal, they hoped to engulf India and then, in turn, subvert the world (Crane, 2002). However, the insurgency was not linked to China. For the most part, 'Nepalese Maoists . . . [were] dismissive of China as a reactionary regime' (Crane, 2002, p. 9). The essence of the insurgents' cause was

> the need to end a 'despotic monarchy', change the 'feudal regime' in Nepal and give a 'voice to the people' . . . land for the landless, jobs for the unemployed, representation and money for the provinces, and an end to the exploitation of labor and discrimination against [lower] caste.
>
> (Crane, 2002, p. 11)

Table 2.3 Brinton's (1965) analysis of Nepal's movements and Maoist insurgency

People's movement 1990		*People's movement 2006*	
Symptoms Economic and political instability (Gellner, 2007; Shakya, 2012; Whelpton, 2005); autocratic *Panchayat* system (Schock, 1999, 2005, emphasis added); worsening condition of marginalised groups (Gellner, 2007; Shakya, 2012; Whelpton, 2005); development failure (Panday, 1999, 2012; Riaz & Basu, 2010)	**Rising fever** Formation of loose Coordination Committee by NCP; United Leftist Front; United National People's Movement; broad-based people participation (Panday, 1999, 2012; Riaz & Basu, 2010)	**Symptoms** Unsettled and unorganised convalescence of 1990 movement itself (Pfaff-Czarnecka, 2004a); Maoist insurgency (Lawoti, 2010; Thapa, 2012); growing economic crisis; Royal massacre; King Gyanendra coup and dispelling parliament in 2005 (Muni, 2012)	**Rising fever** Seven Political Party Alliance; Nepal Democracy Solidarity Group formed in India; 12-point understanding between Maoist and Seven Political Party Alliance; and not least, broad-based people participation (Muni, 2012)
Crisis No significant crisis, as explained by Crane (2002), however royalists were checked, monitored, and controlled by different means	**Convalescence** Establishment of multiparty democracy; Constitutional monarch; Constitution of 1990; General election of 1991 (Whelpton, 2005)	**Crisis** Same as of in the case of 1990 movement	**Convalescence** Declaration of Federal Democratic Republic of Nepal; arrival of United Nations Mission to Nepal and beginning of peace process (Martin, 2012); Interim Constitution (Bhandari, 2014); promulgation of constitution after two constitution assembly elections

In other words, Nepal's long-term structural factors – endemic poverty and horizontal inequality, as well as its lame democracy and inefficient bureaucracy – served as a catalyst for the Maoist insurgency (Brown, 2001; Hutt, 2004; Wallensteen, 2014). Nepal offered a fertile ground for the Maoist revolution, as Crane (2002) observed, 'The countryside . . . [had] been neglected by the governing classes and exploited by absent landlords. There . . . [was] widespread poverty and decreasing hope . . . and . . . [existing] conditions . . . [were] full of despair' (p. 12). The centre of the insurgency was the Far-Western Development Region, which was characterised by deep and abject poverty, polygamy, high birth rates, indentured labour, widespread child labour, and low literacy (Crane, 2002). Above all, while the Maoist insurgency caused heavy losses of lives, infrastructure destruction, and economic slowdown, it also dramatically improved sociopolitical awareness, institutional reforms, and political mobilisation, as shown in Table 2.4. However, despite the people's movements of 1990 and 2006, Nepal's quest for rights, justice, development, and democracy remains tenuous, at best, and a legitimate state (Lake, 2010) and free civil society (Mozaffar, 2010) has yet to materialise.

There is a tug of war between political parties and their leaders, as well as among Nepali citizens, on whether Nepal should embrace an ethnic-centred or democracy-based federalism. While many lower castes and *Janajatis* populations advocate a liberal view of justice with positive discrimination (Rawls, 2009), higher caste groups favour Sen's (2011) capability approach, while the elite holds to a libertarian view centred on rights and entitlements (Nozick, 2013).

Justice for Nepal's most marginalised and vulnerable groups requires deep structural reform (Ake, 1994; Bhandari, 2014; Diamond, 1997) and a release from the stranglehold of self-interested politicians, the caste system, and the redistribution of land and capital concentrated in the hands of a few educated elites (Migdal, 1988; Pfaff-Czarnecka, 2008). Many Nepali scholars and their counterparts across the globe have highlighted that Nepal's current challenges are to develop a stable democratic system, a strong civil society, a strategic approach to policy reform, and a rights-based approach to reduce ethnic cleavages that compromise justice (Bhandari, 2014; Gurung, 2009;

Table 2.4 Cost-benefit analysis of Maoist insurgency

Benefits		Costs	
Sociopolitical awareness		**Human cost**	
Class	Large scale	People killed	Over 10,000
Ethnic/caste	Significant	People disabled, extortion	Thousands
Gender	Significant	Traumatised people	Millions
Political mobilisation		Internal displacement	200,000
Ethnic fronts	Around a dozen	**Infrastructure destruction**	
Youth	Large scale	VDC offices	1369 (35%)
Women	Significant	Schools closed and destroyed	Hundreds
Institutions		Telecommunication towers	105
Traditional	Erosion	Electricity stations	13
Constitution	Flaws identified	Airports	12
Sociopolitical structures	Inequality and injustice exposed	Development projects	318
Service and development		**Political and economic cost**	
Development	Minimal	Civil liberty	Constrained
Social services	Minimal	Political rights	Election delayed
Social justice	Considerable	Violent conflicts	Became culture
People's court	Considerable	Bank robbery	99,766,000
		Extortion of money and food	Large scale
		Economy	Growth inhibited

Source: Adapted from Lawoti (2005, p. 61)

Hangen, 2009; Lawoti, 2012; Panday, 2012; Riaz & Basu, 2010). As Bhandari (2014) argued, Nepal requires the

> systematic, strategic, and forced undertaking demanded by the post-national state . . . to catch up to the developmental aspirations and build the countries to be internally competitive, administratively efficient, and institutionally robust for paving growth and promoting human services development.
>
> (p. 116)

In short, the NCP's democratic and socialist position, as well as several communist parties' communist ideology and nationalism, dominate Nepal's new political narratives. The major difference between the NCP and communist parties revolves around issues of class and status. Nepali communists, including the Communist Party of Nepal (Unified Marxist-Leninist), seek to institutionalise Mao Zedong's doctrine of a populist democracy – a system of government led by the people (proletariat), with representation from other classes. However, a form of demos nationalism that is gaining momentum among DIMM is overshadowing both the NCP and communist parties' political agendas. Equality, rights, and freedom undergird this system.

Thus, in my opinion, Nepal might best be described as a 'hybrid Third World nation' that is in a state of fragile development, its abundant social capital, resilience, and willingness to innovate notwithstanding. It is on the brink of becoming part of the so-called Fourth World by embracing its diverse ethnic and minority groups not currently represented in its emergent nation state (Manuel & Posluns, 1974). Nepal has potential to escape underdevelopment by looking inward and bridging ethnic divisions and social cleavages that block productivity and progress.

Lifestyles, values, and identities: cultural narratives

Cultural narratives represent

> an ontological condition of social life . . . [through which] people construct identities (however multiple and changing) by locating themselves or being located within a repertoire of . . . stories; . . . people make sense of what has happened and is happening to them by attempting to assemble or in some way to integrate these happenings within one or more narratives; and . . . are guided to act in certain ways, and not others, on the basis of the projections, expectations, and memories derived from a multiplicity but ultimately limited repertoire of available social, public, and cultural narratives.
>
> (Somers, 1994, p. 614)

A Nepali lifestyle, value, and identity remain an unfinished project of modernisation and westernisation. Gould (1961) proposed a dynamic relationship between Srinivas' (1956) concept of Sanskritisation – a process by which lower castes gain upward mobility – and the embrace of westernisation by upper caste groups. While more enlightened Nepali people, like the upper caste, embrace Western ways of thinking, they also entrench discriminatory caste practices to keep the hierarchical ordering of society firmly in place. In other words, they strive to maintain their superiority and privileged position by keeping the lower castes at the bottom strata of society.

Though traditional paternalistic practices embedded in caste and linguistic division, and the extended family and arranged marriage system remain firmly entrenched, Nepal's social and structural institutions are changing rapidly, albeit at a slower pace than the rest of the world (Bhusal & Shahi, 2013; Onta & Katherine, 2004; Pandey, Dhakal, Karki, Poudel, & Pradhan, 2013; Whelpton, 2005). Divorce remains rare among Nepali couples, while preference for male children and a belief that women are subordinate to men remain strong in almost all ethnic groups (Whelpton, 2005). Patriarchy pervades family and community life.

The tendency for lower caste groups to adopt upper castes lifestyles and values has led to a rise in the adoption of the Nepali language by non-CHHE people in the hope of greater social inclusion. Further, many castes and *Janajatis* groups tend to follow CHHE group cultures. Many, except Muslims and Christians, now celebrate *Teej*, a festival celebrated mainly by CHHE women to ensure their husbands' longevity and prosperity. High castes, such as Brahmin and Kshatriya, have sought to adopt the culture of the ex-royal and Rana families. It is thus common to observe Brahmin and Kshatriya people communicating within their own groups using the suffix *siyos*, which means ex-royal or alluding to their Rana family connections. *Hajur* has replaced *tapai*, used as a mark of respect for elders.

Yet, Nepal is culturally unique!

Beside these adopted cultural practices, many original social rituals and rhythms remain alive and entrenched from Nepal's high Himalayas to its lowest fringes. In the hills and in the flatlands, where major trade or tourist routes are scarce, the mode of communication continues in its traditional form through folklore, music, and stories. Not only rituals and rhythms but also many of Nepal's languages, in the absence of written script, have relied on oral transmission for generations (Luger & Höivik, 2004). People, irrespective of their religious origins, have a deep sense of reverence for nature. From the Himalayas to the caves, hills, forests, and rivers, all forms of nature are god's creation. Himalayan Buddhists consider the peaks of the Himalayas the 'soul' of the community. Likewise, in the hills and flatlands, people believe the forest is a place of *Vandevta* (god of the forest). Many Nepali people consider nature as a source of power, energy, and livelihoods, as well as threats, which is why they are accustomed to maintaining a safe distance and handling nature with care.

The inherent messages behind these customary practices are to conserve and preserve nature, in ways that western development experts, including foreign social workers, would find it difficult to understand. Nepal was, and continues to be, an agrarian-based economy. Unique agriculture activities, religious festivals, seasonal gatherings, visits to temples and monasteries, and dance and processions are fora through which Nepali people celebrate, share news, and exchange ideas (Downs, 1980; Stevens, 1996). To such rhythms, Högger (1997), echoing Tibetologist Diemberger's (2002) *beseelter landschaft* – landscape charged with spirituality (in Luger & Höivik, 2004) – claimed Nepali people's interaction with their surroundings is an inherent part of their spiritual reality:

> The temple courtyard is a living space, and the landscape is a temple. Both indicate the existence of another, obvious reality above and beyond themselves. This is the essential means of cultural awareness that has become alien to the west.
>
> (Högger, 1997, p. 28)

Nepali people's sense of time differs from that of Westerners. For instance, *bistarai janus* (travel slowly), *bistarai basnus* (sit slowly), *bistrai khanus* (eat slowly), and *bistarai garnus* (perform slowly) typify belief in the philosophical value of pause and reflection (Luger & Höivik, 2004). Other valued practices include planting trees, managing solid waste, harvesting rain water, using solar power (sustainable environment and ecology); raising voices against abuse and discrimination (justice and fairness); volunteering in times of disasters (humanitarian sensitivity); and preventing the slaughtering of animals (animal rights) (Parajuli et al., 2015). The willingness to contribute labour to *nwaran* (celebration of the ninth day of birth), *bihe* (marriage), *bhoj-bhatera* (feast), and *malami* (mourning), that is, sense of communitarianism are long-established traditional social norms. These practices have survived despite westernisation. Although modern organisations, such as youth clubs, non-government organisations (NGOs), community-based organisations (CBOs), and INGOs, and professional networks are transforming these traditions, they remain important sociocultural dynamics in Nepali people's lives.

Moreover, Hinduism, apart from its caste hierarchy, inspires its many followers to practice benevolence and humanism. The concept of *dana* (charity), *dharma* (religion), *karma* (fate), and *moksha* (salvation) are deeply rooted principles in Hinduism and Buddhism, which symbolically contribute to egalitarian welfare practices. Likewise, several verses from Hindu scripts, such as *atithi devo bhava* (a guest is equivalent to God) and *vasudhaiva kuṭumbakam* (the world is one family), typify Nepali hospitality and collective identities rooted in kinship and communitarianism.

Further, Högger (1997) observed that, in Nepali society, two mutually reinforcing processes informed people's knowledge – *padhera* (learning through formal education) and *parera* (learning through experience). Many young Nepali social work graduates trained in a western social work education model might likely question this Nepali tradition. In fact, the literal translation of the word 'social work' into Nepali is *samajik karya* – an activity carried out by volunteers with experiential knowledge built from practice. The rising number of social work graduates and increasing popularity of social work education, mainly in the capital city of Kathmandu, has challenged the concept of *samajik karya*. Professionally trained Nepali social workers struggle to find the correct Nepali terminology for western-style social work in Nepal and remain unaware of the idea of decolonised social work (Gray, Coates, & Yellow Bird, 2008b, 2013c).

Context of social services: state and non-state actors

The Nepali government seeks to address social problems and provide services as a signatory to international human rights and humanitarian charters, treaties, declarations, and conventions (Human Rights Treaty Monitoring Coordination Committee, 2008). The Constitution (GoN, 2015) provides fundamental principles to promote the rights of Nepali peoples, uplift weaker sections of the population, and promote good governance. These include the right to property, equality, social justice, and freedom of religion, as well as proscriptions against untouchability and racial discrimination.

The Social Welfare Council (SWC) under the Ministry of Women, Children, and Social Welfare is a prominent state body charged with social service provision and social development. Its main brief is to coordinate social welfare-oriented institutions and organisations providing social service programs for vulnerable and marginalised sections of society. Under the Social Welfare Act 1992, the SWC is responsible for services related to the welfare of children, older people, and people with disabilities

(GoN, 1992a). Further, it seeks to protect and promote the rights and participation of women in social development. Its roles include rehabilitation for those who are socially, economically, and politically disadvantaged and unable to integrate into mainstream of society. The SWC also oversees the welfare of the so-called 'backward' communities and groups in Nepal (GoN, 1992a). Further, it takes responsibility for the monitoring and evaluation of the non-governmental social organisations in the country (see Chapter 3). To date, however, its success has been minimal (Gurung, 2009). Consequently, social services in Nepal are ineffective, poor in quality, expensive, and discriminatory. INGOs and internationally funded internal NGOs do much of the social development work.

However, the government has introduced legislation and social security programs to improve the livelihoods of Nepali people and protect the most vulnerable sections of the population (see Figure 2.5). Several acts and regulations protect the interests of specific groups, such as children, women, older people, and people with disabilities (GoN, 2012a). In keeping with international development policy, the state adopts a neoliberal New Public Management approach to facilitate the active involvement of non-state actors, such as CBOs, NGOs, INGOs, humanitarian organisations (HOs), and religious institutions in service delivery. There are many layers of NGOs from national to

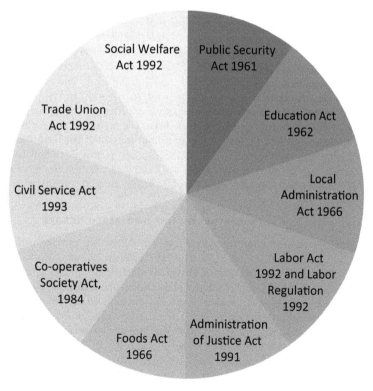

Figure 2.5 Nepali social legislations

Source: Adapted from GoN (2012a)

regional, urban, and rural CBOs (Tanaka, 2011). They work across a wide spectrum from HIV and AIDS to child welfare and community and rural – social, economic, educational, and environmental – development, as well as providing services for people with disabilities, women, children, and young people (SWC, 2014b). The Ninth Five-Year Plan (1997–2002) and Self-Governance Act (1999) officially recognised the role of NGOs in national development (Tanaka, 2011). Moreover, the Interim Three-Year Plan (2007/8–2009/10) perceived NGOs as a vehicle for the rights-based empowerment of excluded groups, such as *Dalits, Janajatis*, and women (GoN, 2008). Along with multilateral and bilateral agencies, INGOs are major stakeholders in social development programs and activities in Nepal (see Chapter 3). Importantly, INGOs provide employment to social work graduates and, therefore, constitute an important focus for this book.

To obtain community sanction and accredited professional status, Nepali social workers need to engage in a process of decolonisation to make it locally and culturally relevant. In terms of the National Directive Act 1961, the SWC is the only relevant mainline institution that can make recommendations to the cabinet *vis-à-vis* the professional status of social work in Nepal. Hence, the roles and responsibilities of the SWC are of interest to social workers, since a legitimate, socially sanctioned social work profession would likely fall within its ambit.

Conclusion

This chapter has outlined Nepal's history; its geographic, social, and political complexities; the caste system that undergirds its social structure; its ethnic diversity; and the unique cultures and traditions of its peoples. It is a country poised at the dawn of a new democracy for ethnic representation and rights-based fairness and justice for all. Rather than ignoring or dismissing Nepali dynamics – including history, social, and political crises, and unique lifestyle – as an awkward past, it is important to centralise these into Nepali studies, especially in social work education. The following chapter discusses INGOs and their role as change agents in Nepali development.

Chapter 3

International non-government organisations and Nepali development

A place for Nepali social workers to engage

As a modern nation state, Nepal evokes ambiguous sentiments. It has become a fertile ground for national and international anthropologists, political rationalists, intrepid explorers, adventure tourists, and development specialists. Despite its experience of never having been colonised, its abundant natural resources, and numerous movements for socioeconomic and political change, it remains one of the least developed nations in the world. Since the second half of the 20th century, international communities, through transnational and national NGOs, have treated the country as an exotic space in which to dance with Nepali development (Collier, 2013). This chapter critically examines the involvement of INGOs in Nepal's development – their contribution and the progress made.

Nepal has witnessed never-ending setbacks because of the nation's snail-pace development, contentious political agenda, and poor service delivery. Leaders, technocrats, and legislators are far more concerned about their own political interests than guaranteeing human rights, meeting development needs, and valuing the principles of democracy, inclusiveness, representation, self-determination, and diversity. Their political agenda manifests injustice and intolerance as these Nepali authorities ignore international human rights and development agendas.

Historically, since its inception as a modern state in 1768, Nepal has been an independent and sovereign country unable to 'provide predictable, recognizable, systematized methods of adjudicating disputes and regulating both the norms and the prevailing mores' (Rotberg, 2010, p. 3). Its polities neither engage nor enable its citizens to participate fully and freely in the political and social milieu. Its deteriorating services and infrastructure are the result of its institutional fragilities, fractured across its history by the domination of the Shah Dynasty and Rana regime, and contesting political parties. Destabilising forces stem from the country's ethnic antagonism, administrative stagnation, elite-led decision-making, and the external influence of China and India. Nepal has never shown itself to be sensitive to its people's development needs. Its ruling elites have not exhibited the political will to guarantee social development, as reflected in successive development measures, such as the Human Development Index (UNDP, 2013), Corruption Perception Index (Transparency International, 2014), Freedom of the World Report (Freedom House, 2015), and the Amnesty International Report 2014/15: The State of the World's Human Rights (Amnesty International, 2015).

In a situation where the state apparatus rarely revisits its role in social development, Nepal has performed surprisingly well in its progress toward the Millennium Development Goals 2015 due largely to the presence of INGOs in the country (GoN & UN

Nepal, 2013). There are 211 INGOs and 39763 NGOs affiliated with SWC (SWC 2015a, 2015b). The GoN and UNDP (2014) reported that these organisations collectively set 'a federal development agenda that facilitates a multi-pronged approach to raising productive ability which can ensure sustainable human development' (p. viii). Moreover, INGOs set a crucial development platform funding several government and non-government organisations and collaborating with local counterparts in development interventions.

Metaphysics of, and definitional challenges to, INGOs

Bloodgood and Schmitz (2013) believe scholarship on INGOs is difficult due to the lack of a commonly shared definition, problems in tracking their history, and the absence of empirical methodologies to explain their activities. INGOs, as global actors, are visible from New York to the least developed centres of Asia and Africa. Their goals are to promote development, enhance good governance, sustain democracy, and advocate for an egalitarian society. Yet, it is difficult to define INGOs because of their polymorphic nature. Although they collectively serve humanitarian goals, influenced by various international development policies and agenda, they exhibit diverse interests and wide-ranging views of development. Each INGO has a focus or foci, from environmental to health, child welfare, refugee, and women's issues. Hence, INGOs usually define themselves in terms of their area of focus and nature of the work they do or assistance they render. Their philosophy and activities notwithstanding, INGOs come under constant scrutiny and criticism for focusing on technical solutions and measurable outcomes. Though their philosophy reflects a humanitarian ethos, and contemporary development policy embodies a focus on human development and people's participation therein, on-the-ground implementation frequently overlooks local cultural contingencies and country-specific needs and does not engage with structural change or giving people a voice and representation in local politics (Fujikura, 2001).

Terminology

INGOs are international non-government organisations that have been variously referred to as 'not-for-profit organisations', 'non-government organisations', 'development organisations', 'private voluntary organisations', 'international good governance organisations', 'global civil society organisations', 'global public service contractors', and 'global watchdogs' (Korten, 1990; Macdonald, 1994; Murdie, 2014; Robinson, 1994).

History

Boli and Thomas (1999a) tracked the history of INGOs from 1875 onwards through three major phases:

1   *The early influence of philanthropy and ethical notion of giving beyond the family*: Often influenced by religious and charitable activities, the prime motif of early international organisations was support to fellow peoples.
2   *Vicissitudes of World War I and II in Europe*: The universalistic philanthropic ethos changed dramatically post–World War II as economic reconstruction and development assumed dominance.

3   *Emergence of world culture and transnational structures,* such as the UN, that promoted internationalisation and enabled INGOs to assume dominance in all spheres of development through global agreements and the growth of a human rights culture.

Ideology of INGOs

Depending on their diverse purposes, INGOs embrace broader ideologies relating to development, foreign aid, poverty alleviation, humanitarian assistance, disaster management and recovery, child well-being, and human rights. Thus, discussions on the ideologies or humanitarian values that motivate INGOs in their search for a better quality of life for people affected by poverty, natural disasters, civil conflict, HIV and AIDS, human trafficking, child labour, and so on, necessarily involve engaging in broader discourses on the relationship between development, foreign aid, and poverty alleviation (Fujikura, 2001). Many have explained, for example Griffin (2009), Portes (1997), and Rankin (2001), that development has more to do with embedding neoliberal economic growth models and encouraging favourable conditions for international trade than with poverty alleviation or improving the quality of people's lives. There are debates on whether foreign aid is an effective way of facilitating development and poverty alleviation. There are myriad accounts of corruption whereby aid does not reach the beneficiaries for whom it is intended and debates on whether aid is best dispensed through national governments or NGOs. Generally, however, INGOs envision a world of porous boundaries and global citizenship, one where human rights, social justice, a representative and participatory democracy, a neoliberal economic system, strong national and local governance, a solid infrastructure, mutual accountability and partnership, and law and order pertains; that is, their vision is Western. Boli and Thomas (1999b) believe that a global development perspective rooted in global rationalism, volunteerism, and institutional theory motivates INGOs. They see development as an invention of modernisation and globalisation and the historical narrative of progressivism (or modernising development).

Global rationalism perceives the world as a unified entity with moral authority stamped on world society, world culture, world citizens, and the world polity. It leads to a form of global governance that not only presumes 'oneness of place and time . . . solely or essentially material or techno-economic . . . [but] also cultural and political [harmony]' (Thomas, 2007, p. 37). It gives rise to a global consciousness comprising cognitive schema, models of authority, and rational development goals that transcend local cultures and contexts (Douglas, 1996):

> World culture is composed of categories of things (endangered species, industrial zones, legal contracts, profits, nation-states, individuals), identities (ethnic, national, religious, gender), and models of action and organization (development, democracy, research, planning) that are pervasive throughout the world across all sorts of borders.
> (Thomas, 2007, p. 37)

This world culture connects Nepal with the external world. Even the case of introducing professional social work education and practice in Nepal is the product of world culture and globalisation. Given that social work's own international institutions are themselves INGOs, they too envisage Nepal as a market for social work expansion, for bringing the values and mission of social work to Nepal's diverse cultures, and for embedding social work education within their expansionist-imperialist frame. Social work's internationalising discourse makes it possible for bearers of social work degree from all over the world – as world citizens – to practice in Nepal, bringing with them their social work ideology of professionalism.

This global rationalism brought modernising INGOs to Nepal with the promise of development. This too is premised on the goals of world 'peace, justice, progress, development, effective democratic governance, [and human] health, and well-being' (Thomas, 2007, p. 38). INGOs bring scientific advances in knowledge and technology, democratic governance structures, and neoliberal models of economic growth premised on a rational moral order that privileges a form of progressive, modernising development (Fujikura, 2001). Nepal's fragile bureaucracy and governance structures, lacking as they are in financial and technical expertise, created an easy passage for INGOs that have mushroomed in Nepal (see Figure 3.1).

The idea of world citizenship, though seemingly diffuse and abstract, is strongly egalitarian and rests on individuals enjoying the same basic rights and duties, entitlements and responsibilities, and accessibility to resources sitting alongside institutional accountability, irrespective of context. As Boli and Thomas (1999a) wrote,

> World citizenship is the institutional endowment of authority and agency on individuals. It infuses each individual with the authority to pursue particularistic interests, preferably in organizations, while also authorizing individuals to promote collective goods defined in largely standardized ways.
>
> (p. 40)

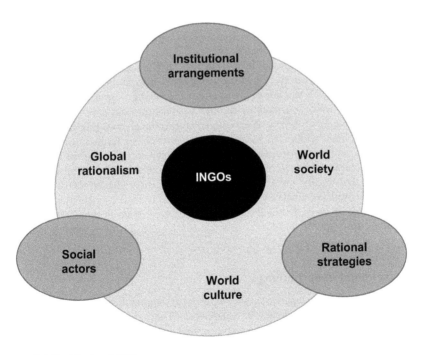

Figure 3.1 Positioning INGOs

A world polity – global civil society enjoying human rights, justice, fairness, and self-determination – that keeps the state, market, and regional and international agencies honest through political participation and activism frames this world citizenship. Too often, however, the opposite pertains with critics believing INGOs serve the world market, state apparatus, and political parties rather than the world polity or civil society (Fujikura, 2001). Generally, however, INGOs encourage universalism and call for open participation for their members to accelerate universal well-being. In short, they are platforms for like-minded people who view development through a prism of global rationalism and volunteerism (Boli & Thomas, 1999a).

Epistemology: INGO discourse

INGO discourse reflects a faith in scientific advancement and technological development, in rational models of economic growth, and in rational policy and decision-making within a democratic system of governance. It is an inherently Western epistemology based on an overarching belief in modernising, scientific development, economic growth, and human rights. This epistemological bent has spawned the trickle-down effect, rational choice theory, and neoliberal structural adjustment. There is, too, however, a humanistic side to development seen in its self-help, community development ethos and valuing of equality, solidarity, cooperation, and participation (Bongartz & Dahal, 1996). This human rights and social justice discourse, with its focus on human and social development, sits alongside economic growth models of development (Fujikura, 2001; Panday, 1999, 2011, 2012; Pigg, 1992, 1993; Shrestha, 1997, 2000; Shrestha et al., 2008).

Examining INGO discourse through various theoretical and disciplinary lenses leads to various understandings and interpretations of development, as reflected in political science, economics, and sociological and development studies perspectives. From a critical perspective, development is a product of colonisation and modernisation and as a strategy for globalisation to embed neoliberal economics in the Global South.

From within INGO discourse, international organisations promote social development and social protection working through national governments, non-government organisations, and civil society. National and international laws, guidelines, and procedures bind them, while civil societies may or may not be limited in the same way. Nevertheless, national governments, INGOs, and civil society collectively endeavour to promote and protect sociopolitical development and national security. It is difficult to separate civil society and INGOs as both emerge from shared platforms, such as development, welfare, advocacy, and political activism. To the extent that they share Western historical roots, Duffield (2014) suggests, in more recent times, they are moving within the 'logic of the North's new security regime' (p. 16) to prevent attacks on Western values.

Philosophical underpinnings

Whether they are agents, analysts, or activists in the development domain, INGOs employ several standard terms to demarcate their work. They are voluntary, not-for-profit, non-government, non-state, third sector, or civil society organisations, and, in more recent times, social entrepreneurs or social economy organisations. They are authoritative, legitimate bodies within the development arena through their internationally visible and locally significant symbolic, moral, and material *episteme*. Strong normative positions ground them, though empirical effectiveness studies have become increasing important within results accountability, evidence-based development models. Although they emerged at the first World Congress of International Association and the London Conference of the International Law Association, both held in 1910, international social organisations were not new to world politics even then (Murdie, 2014). They were already working against slavery in the 18th and 19th centuries (Keck & Sikkink, 1998), with their vision, mission, and interventions rooted in ancient philosophy on the relationship between the state and its peoples that continued to evolve through the medieval and modern eras.

St Augustine's naturalistic philosophy perceived a naturalness to civil society born of human nature and human beings' natural desire for association, that is, their social natures. We might see the roots of INGOs here in the 'association of men [sic] united by a common set of interests and . . . sense of justice' (Robertson, 1993, pp. 29–30), presaging organisations of like-minded actors that, in medieval times, centred on individual rights to property, liberty, and freedom of association. The philosophy of St Thomas Aquinas, who saw it as a function of human nature to pursue the common good, reflects this naturalism; human beings were naturally inclined to desire harmony and social order (Bongartz & Dahal, 1996). There was little awareness then that these ideas applied mainly to men, whites, and wealthy elites or that guilds and associations represented some interests at the expense of others.

The rise of liberalism and the social contract in Locke's *Sovereign* (Franklin, 1978; Locke, 1821), Hobbes' *Political Sovereign* (Baumgold, 1988), and Rousseau's *General Will* (Rousseau, 1968) embedded the values of individual freedom, justice, democracy, and minimal state involvement in social matters. Kant embodied this liberal sentiment in his idea that real freedom and enlightenment could only exist when legislative power expressed the united will of the people (Bongartz & Dahal, 1996).

However, Durkheim (1997) rejected the notion of a social contract in favour of association as an essential means to maintain social solidarity, cohesion, and integration. Bongartz and Dahal (1996) related social solidarity to global rationalism, social cohesion to global citizenship, and social integration to the blurring of national boundaries in the globalised world. INGOs reflected the right to organise and decide without interference from institutional, bureaucratic, technological, and industrial arrangements. Habermas (1987), for example, saw INGOs as cosmopolitan organisations separate from the state and corporate sectors (Bongartz & Dahal, 1996).

At a meta-theoretical level, INGOs have been seen through the lens of *inter alia* liberal cosmopolitanism (democracy and legitimation), rational-constructivism (ideas, norms, and policy), critical constructivism, post-structuralism, and neo-Gramscianism (power, privilege, knowledge, and resistance). The critical perspective of Marxist and Gramscian thought sees global social organisations as evolving out of production and commerce, encapsulating 'the totality of economic, social, and political realities of [a] capitalist order' (Shah, 2008, p. 7). For Gramsci, these organisations, positioned between state and market elites, perpetuated the hegemony of capitalist sociocultural and moral values. Others, like Dewey and Habermas, however, saw them as organs of democracy (Cochran, 2010); though Hudock (1999) claimed INGOs were agents of 'proxy, rather than true democracy' (p. 13). This is perhaps why, after six decades of INGOs engagement in Nepal, there have been no tangible impacts in developing and sustaining democratic governance. However, examinations in terms of Eastern schools of thought highlight that the history of voluntary organisation in Nepal is as old as the society itself (Carapico, 2000; Dhakal, 2006, 2007). It can be seen in traditional volunteer (voluntary) organisations and activities created even before the unification of Nepal in 1768 (Bhattachan, 2000; Chand, 1991), based on the values of trust, and organised around *guthi*, *pati-pauwa* (shelter), *dharm bhakari* (local grain bank), *parma* (labour exchange system), and *dhikur* (savings or credit). Dhakal (2007) noted the number of volunteer organisations grounded in Eastern philosophy was believed to be as many as 200,000 in Nepal. However, he noted too that, due to their miniscule and scattered nature and uncoordinated *modus operandi*, 'their roles have been under-explored' (p. 63).

Teleology: purpose and mission of INGOs

From a teleological perspective, the significance and legitimacy of INGOs depend on their values, purpose, and mission. In post-war development, they became identified with the spread of Western capitalism and efforts of Western governments to stem the tide of communism and ensure the security of liberal Western political economics. The UNDP (1994) reflected this purpose in its claim that INGOs ensured a secure society by freeing the world from 'want' and 'fear'. Boli and Thomas (1999a) claimed they did this through voluntary action, their rational voluntaristic authority, and philosophy of universalism and rational progress:

> Almost all INGOs originate and persist via voluntary action by individual actors. They have explicit, rationalized goals. They operate under strong norms of open membership and democratic decision-making. They seek, in a general sense, to spread 'progress' throughout the world: to encourage safer and more efficient technical systems, more powerful knowledge structures, better care of the body, friendly competition and fair play.
>
> (p. 34)

INGOs' value-laden universalistic framework was seen to knit interested or like-minded individuals and nations across the globe together around particular interests (Robertson, 1992, 1994). For example, Save the Children, which works in more than 120 countries, including Nepal, seeks to promote and protect children worldwide. However, more than this, powerful INGOs, like the major international financial institutions, control the tide of development through international policies and charters that are binding upon nations and aid-contingent, conditional development funding that shapes practices in similar ways across widely diverse contexts. Hence INGOs, with their headquarters in different parts of the world, have been able to secure a unique place in Nepal and exert a strong influence on the country's policies, programs, and services.

Technology

Technological development has been a major focus of INGOs involved in development worldwide and became synonymous with modernisation and progress. The development of computer technology in the information age has connected people across the world in unprecedented ways, allowing for the standardisation of practices within a globalised world. Technology assists in the design, development, and implementation of policies and programs (operational functions) and the promotion of rights-based policies

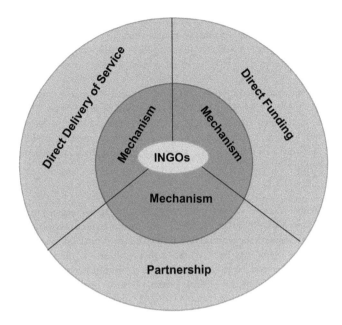

Figure 3.2 Control mechanism

and practices through state and non-state agencies (advocacy functions) (Finnemore & Sikkink, 1998; Keck & Sikkink, 1998; Murdie, 2014; Murdie & Davis, 2012). INGOs, like Amnesty International and Human Rights Watch, act as watchdogs 'naming and shaming' and 'shaming and blaming' groups or nations that violate human rights. In Nepal's regime change from a monarchy to a republic in 2008, advocacy INGOs used both 'shaming and blaming' and carrot-and-stick strategies (Hafner-Burton, 2008; Schepers, 2006) to force the king to step down. Murdie (2014) identified three main mechanisms by which INGOs exerted control – service delivery, funding, and partnership (see Figure 3.2). Other means include policymaking, program evaluation, and outcome measurement within recent results-accountability frameworks. Here technologies include poverty reduction strategy papers, national development plans, and sustainable development goals. These control mechanisms tie local NGOs in endless reporting with INGOs often playing a mentoring and monitoring role. Often, reporting mechanism involve complex procedures and processes that have spawned development consultants and consultancies, think tanks, workshops, and seminars, and research centres to report on, and increase, aid effectiveness.

INGOs in Nepal

Emergence of INGOs in Nepal

INGOs have received significant attention from scholars and researchers in Nepal (Bhattachan, 1999, 2000; Chand, 1991; Dhakal, 2006, 2007; Fujikura, 2001; Panday,

1999, 2011, 2012; Pigg, 1992, 1993; Shrestha, 1997; Shrestha et al., 2008). The growth of INGOs began following the country's first experience of democracy in 1951, after over a century of Herculean, feudalistic Ranas rule. The Ranas regime purposefully restricted Nepal's exposure to the outside world fearing this would hamper its autocracy. As Crane (2002) noted,

> In 1951 a national uprising, inspired by the recent independence of India, threw out the Ranas and restored the King to a position of real power. The King, 'conservative' in the sense that he sought to protect what was best in Nepal but change that which would otherwise be swept away by the currents of History, ended Nepal's self-imposed isolation and began an experiment with democracy, which in many ways is still in process.
>
> (p. 2)

In the post-Rana regime, several externally initiated social organisations emerged, which were inspired by Christian missions, such as the United Mission and Helvetas, both of which facilitated the emergence of NGOs in Nepal during the 1950s. The United Mission to Nepal has been working in health and community development since 1954, while Helvetas Nepal initiated projects to empower farmers from the hill communities. These remain the core activities of these organisations to the present day. Some of the first INGOs working in Nepal, such as the British Medical Trust, International Nepal Fellowship, and International Netherland Funds were extensions of projects operating from India. When INGOs first entered to Nepal, the literacy rate was about four percent and there was no infrastructure, industry, or social development (Dahal, 2002). These early INGOs faced the challenge of unstable politics, extreme underdevelopment, and a lack of trained human resources which, to some extent, remains the case even now. Between the late 1950s and early 1960s, the Swiss Red Cross and New Zealand Red Cross Societies started providing financial support to Nepal's Red Cross Society, while in 1957 Save the Children UK formally extended technical support to the Nepal Children's Organisation of which the then queen Ratna Rajya Lakshmi was a patron.

In 1960, the *Panchayat* system banned all political parties and centralised power in the King for the next 30 years. Its strict regulation of civil society slowed the growth of INGOs during this period. In the 1970s, however, a few INGOs in the Himalayan Kingdom, as it was then referred to, came with their mission to uplift the population from socioeconomic suffering. They included the British Red Cross Society, Swedish Red Cross, League of Red Cross Society, and Oxfam. Today Oxfam engages in broadbased activities in the field of disaster recovery, food security, humanitarian aid, social inclusion, and gender empowerment, among others (Chand, 2002).

In 1977, the Social Service National Co-ordination Act (also known as *Samajik Sewa Ain*) was established to regulate NGOs in Nepal. This encouraged many INGOs to involve local NGOs in their development activities. As result, the largest international organisations, including Care International, Action Aid, Lutheran World Services, and Save the Children USA, signed an agreement with the Social Service National Co-ordination Committee, and, by the end of the 1980s, there were already 49 INGOs working in diverse sectors across the country (Chand, 2002).

Despite their ongoing funding of local NGOs, relationships between international and local NGOs have sometimes been fractious. In 1991, INGOs became a hot topic in Nepal, as local NGO leaders questioned their policies and approaches and demanded that they limit their operations to the institutional and professional development of their local counterparts; also, rather than direct engagement with local communities, they demanded that they leave the implementation of action plans to their local partners. This clamour for power significantly influenced the government, which resulted in the establishment of the Social Welfare Act in 1992 to regulate non-government organisations. This remains the legislative framework governing INGOs in the country, too. In this way, the 1990s brought important debates on the relationship between the Global North and the Global South, and critiques of the vested interests of Northern INGOs in Nepal.

Fisher (1997) noted the growth of INGOs across the globe, and in Nepal, was linked to broad sociopolitical and economic changes in modern societies and, more recently, neoliberal global governance. As flexible humanitarian and advocacy organisations (Lewis & Kanji, 2009), INGOs were able to accommodate diverse actors, ideologies, and contexts by providing a safe space for popular movements to counter modern forms of imperialism and oppression with their empowerment rhetoric (Clarke, 1998), while adhering to market-driven practices to restrict state intervention and foster privatisation (DeMars, 2005). Either way, their goal was to transform the lives of vulnerable and marginalised populations in the Global South. How they did this has been a matter of some contention, especially from the Left. For example, Temple (1997) claimed that, by perpetuating Western capitalist values and norms, they destroyed local economies and cultures founded on interdependence and social solidarity. Hence, INGOs in Nepal have been criticised as 'come-and-go organisations' (referring to their short-term intervention), part of the 'dollar business' (referring to their US roots), 'evangelist' (referring to their faith-based links), 'imperialist' (referring to their hegemonous nature), purveyors of 'development romanticism' and 'dependency creators' (referring to their idealistic view of progress). In short, they were neoliberal institutions imposing a political economy on Nepal's underdeveloped state.

Defining the status of INGOs in Nepal

As already shown, most INGOs are defined in terms of their purpose, though few have a sole purpose, and many perform multiple functions. Care Nepal, for example, focuses on women's empowerment, natural resource management, and better livelihoods for Nepali people. INGOs have also been defined in terms of the services they render or the ethos driving them. For example, faith-based INGOs, especially those inclined to Christianity, have an evangelical mission beyond service rendering to spread their philosophy of how people should live (Spair & Moser, 2007). Increasingly, however, INGOs have a hybrid identity, fulfilling multiple functions and purposes, their 'rights-based' ethos notwithstanding. Murdie (2014) idealistically identified the following defining features of INGOs:

1 They involve individuals with shared goals, values, and actions.
2 They are independent and autonomous agents of civil society.
3 They are not-for-profit and employ market mechanisms to ensure their sustainability.
4 They are non-political and do not support political parties, though they engage in political action to defend human rights and pursue social justice.
5 They work transnationally, employing similar policies, programs, and practices in diverse contexts.

6   Most function legitimately and are registered with national bodies that authorise their operations and activities.

In terms of Nepal's Project Agreement Guidelines (SWC, 2014a), INGOs are defined in terms of their legal, functional, financial, and structural-operational status.

Legal status

The SWC within the Ministry of Women, Children, and Social Welfare registers all INGOs operating in Nepal in terms of the Social Welfare Act (GoN, 1992a). It provides legal sanction for the development activities of INGOs working in Nepal through its compulsory affiliation policy that regards them as government partners rather than autonomous operators. The Project Agreement Guidelines (SWC, 2014a) require all INGOs to contribute to national policy and government programs; engage in balanced developmental activities in terms of gender, geography, and population distribution; ensure financial transparency and social accountability; submit regular progress reports to the SWC; and not allow total administrative costs to exceed 20 percent on any project. Hence, though INGOs are autonomous, their work is highly regulated in Nepal.

Functional status

INGOs carry out broad-based development activities and contribute to national policies and programs, economic growth, and democratic practices. Nepal's unstable politics and weak governance structures have left it heavily reliant on INGOs to address matters of public concern. As Weisbord (1988) explained, being not-for-profit organisations, INGOs are a viable alternative for the supply of non-marketised public goods in the 'public interest'; they are the face of 'public policy' serving Nepali people through poverty-alleviation programs, infrastructure development, and social service provision. They offer an efficient and effective means of delivering goods and services and creating social capital, since they foster 'trust, norms, and networks, that can improve the efficiency of society by facilitating co-ordinated actions' (Putnam, Leonardi, & Nanetti, 1994, p. 167).

Financial status

The UN system of national accounting categorises economic activities into non-profit, non-financial, financial, government, and household categories (United Nations, International Monetary Fund, European Commission, World Bank, & Organisation for Economic Co-operation and Development, 2009). Being non-profit organisations, INGOs receive their income from members, donors, and supporters. They generate significant funds for humanitarian projects and offer financial hope for many Nepali people.

Structural-operational status

According to Salamon and Anheir (1997), INGOs in Nepal share five key characteristics. They are:

1   *Organised*: They are highly bureaucratic institutions that engage in systematic and regular planning, budgeting, monitoring, evaluation, and reporting.

2   *Private*: An autonomous governing board determines and oversees their activities.
3   *Not-for-profit*: They distribute their funds through their mission, programs, and
     activities to uplift the lives of targeted beneficiaries.
4   *Self-governing*: They control and determine their activities and intervention pro-
     cesses and decide on the issues they address, the locations in which they work, and
     the beneficiaries they serve.
5   *Voluntary*: Though they employ large numbers of people, they encourage volun-
     tary participation in their intervention processes, especially at the grassroots level.

In addition, INGOs are:

6   Local: Though they take part in global governance, they operate in local cultural
     contexts. As Nepal is multicultural, multilingual, and multiethnic nation, INGOs
     working in the country cannot bypass peoples' cultural frameworks. Their sensitivity
     to adapt to Nepali context has legitimised their activities in Nepali communities.

In 2014, the Association of International NGOs (AIN) reported that about 50
INGOs entered Nepal during the Maoist insurgency (1996–2006) known as the People's War or Maoist rebellion (von Einsiedel, Malone, & Pradhan, 2012a, 2012b; Hutt,
2004; Lawoti, 2012; Lawoti & Pahari, 2010; Panday, 2012); most were activist INGOs.
SWC (2015a) reported that 211 INGOs from 26 countries were registered operating
in Nepal (see Figure 3.3). The majority were from the USA (n = 62) followed by the
UK (n = 34). European INGOs also have a presence and cover almost all geographical territories. INGOs from Japan (n = 10), Canada (n = 7), and South Korea (n = 7)
followed by Australia (n = 6), Netherlands (n = 6), Belgium (n = 5), and Denmark
(n = 5) are emerging in the country. SWC (2015a) data shows that the countries with
high a Human Development Index have more INGOs in Nepal than those with lower
indices. Surprisingly, Nepal's two neighbours, India and China, have only three and
two INGOs respectively, despite their dominance in Nepali politics.

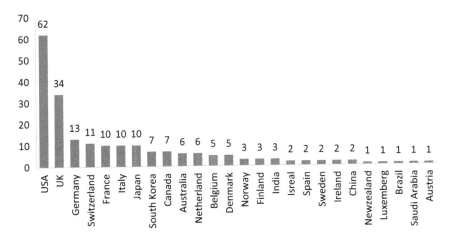

Figure 3.3 INGOs registered with the Social Welfare Council

Source: Adapted from SWC (2015a)

Activities of INGOs in Nepal

In his study of INGOs, Chand (2002) found INGOs' main operations involved technical and financial support. Rather than provide direct services, most contributed to building the organisational capacity of local humanitarian and development NGOs and funded local NGOs, CBOs, and government projects, collaborating with them to implement, monitor, and evaluate programs. Most had limited direct engagement with beneficiaries at the grassroots level. Though this accorded maximum autonomy to local partner NGOs, it also opened the door for the misuse of funds to serve vested interests. Most of the 39,763 NGOs registered with the SWC were heavily dependent on INGOs funding. AIN (2014) reported that INGOs spent 22 billion rupees in 2014, approximately 8–10 percent of Nepal's total foreign aid budget, through their local partners. Yet, despite ongoing capacity-building projects, people's livelihoods continued to fall below global poverty standards and sustainability remains an ongoing issue with few local NGOs becoming independent and able to operate without INGOs support.

Chand (2002) also found that most began their work in collaboration with government agencies or line ministries as a rite of passage through the government's lengthy bureaucratic procedures. Once they had established their legitimacy, they moved into 'long-term local partnerships', working in collaboration with local organisations familiar with the needs and territories of targeted projects and local actors who had a strong relationship with their beneficiaries. The flexibility of these local organisations made for enhanced efficiency and accountability. However, Chand (2002) found that this lack of 'red tapeism', as he put it, was a double-edged sword as some NGOs were involved in partisan politics and used INGOs' funding to buy votes for their chosen political parties. To deal with this problem, INGOs developed a partnership model in which beneficiary groups were involved as members or promoters of local projects.

Governance of INGOs in Nepal

As already outlined, INGOs are granted legal status through the SWC. Table 3.1 summarises the minimum guidelines on the registration, financing, operation, coordination, and monitoring of INGOs in Nepal. Other legal norms relating to INGO activities in Nepal include the Society Registration Act (GoN, 1977), National Directive Act (GoN, 1961), Foreign Exchange (Regulation) Act (GoN, 1962a), Village Development Committee Act (GoN, 1992b), and Local Self-Governance Act (GoN, 1999).

Despite these myriad regulations, a World Bank (2003) study on financial accountability found Nepal's INGOs governance mechanisms required improvement. Most INGOs associated directly with line ministries bypassed the SWC making the real accounting of INGOs performance and expenditure difficult to estimate. Second, SWC's strict bureaucratic procedures and limited resources were unequal to the task of monitoring INGOs financial and banking transactions. Third, the SWC was itself in need of organisational development and capacity building; it did not have enough employees and those who were employed lacked adequate skills and resources to monitor the registered 39,763 NGOs and 211 INGOs. Finally, yet importantly, the SWC committee itself lacked accountability and freedom from party political interference. This related directly to its composition in terms of the Social Welfare Act. It comprised a committee of 19 members chaired by the Minister for Women, Children, and Social Welfare. Ten members were 'social work' nominees and eight were representatives from

Table 3.1 NGO and INGO governance measures

Social Welfare Act 1992	*Project Agreement Guidelines 2014*
• **This act restructured the Social Service National Co-ordination Council 1977.** • **Discusses the provisions to facilitate, coordinate, monitor, evaluate local and international non-government organisations.** • **Acts as a mediator between the government of Nepal and non-government organisations.** • **Functions to advise the government to regulate and formulate social welfare and social service policies.** • **Enhances competencies of non-government organisations.** • **Mobilises national and international non-government organisations support and activities.**	• This is the implementing document of Social Welfare Act 1992. • Broadly discusses nature, coordination, participation, funding, and monitoring and evaluation of non-government organisation. • Advises non-government organisations to focus on the most marginalised and vulnerable populations and geographical areas of Nepal. • Emphasises partnerships with local government and non-government bodies. • Argues to contribute to broader national development policies and programs. • Promotes gender sensitive and population proportionate developmental activities. • Checks the effectiveness and transparency of non-government organisations. • Organises reporting and documentation of non-government organisations. • Facilitates and takes legal actions in the case of non-governmental organisations' abuse of authorities. • Controls the flow of expatriates and administrative costs of any non-government organisations. • Strongly advises non-government organisations to maintain their financial activities in any commercial banks of Nepal.

Source: Adapted from GON (1992a) and SWC (2014a)

the National Planning Commission (NPC), House of Representatives, and Ministries of Home Affairs, Local development, Finance, Health, and Education and Culture. The 'social workers' on the committee were people involved in formal or informal voluntary activities and did not necessarily have a social work qualification.

An initiative is underway to improve NGO effectiveness in Nepal. With the help of the World Bank (2003), in 2002, the SWC proposed a Draft Bill on Non-Governmental Social Development Organizations (NGSDOs) that has yet to be passed. Some key features of the Bill are:

• A broader concept of 'social development' rather than 'social welfare'.
• Renaming of NGO to NGSDO.
• Restructured Social Development Council (SDC) comprising 40 members chaired by the Prime Minister instead of the Minister of Women, Children, and Social Welfare and an Executive Committee comprising eight members overseeing the SDC's management and administrative functions.
• Regulation of all forms of foreign assistance or aid, including that from foreign governments, INGOs, and foreign nationals.

- A work permits system for INGO employees.
- Tripartite agreements between INGOs, government line ministries, and the SDC for INGOs working in direct partnership with government.
- Power to seize or freeze unapproved flows of foreign funds.
- Coordination of INGO, NGO or NGSDO, and local CBO activity by mobilising international funding.

(World Bank, 2003)

However, many of these powers already pertained in the Social Welfare Act of 1992. Rather than a new Bill, the SWC needed to be resourced to implement the existing policy framework.

Development planning and INGOs' engagement in Nepal

Though one of the oldest sovereign, independent states, Nepal's snail-paced development and relatively recent transition to democracy has made it one of the least developed nations in the world, this despite decades of development planning as follows:

- *First Five-Year Plan (1956–1961)*: Infrastructure, transport, and communication were a major focus followed by agriculture, including village development and irrigation. The plan was not well-conceived and only two-thirds of the budget was spent (GoN, 1956; Savada, 1993).
- *Second Three-Year Plan (1962–1965)*: Again infrastructure (transportation and communication) received priority followed by industry, tourism, and social services. Once again, the government failed to spend the budgeted amount (GoN, 1962b; Savada, 1993).
- *Third Five-Year Plan (1965–1970)*: There was an increased involvement of local *panchayat* in the continuing focus on transport, communications, and industrial and agricultural development (GoN, 1965; Savada, 1993).
- *Fourth Five-Year Plan (1970–1975)*: Though the third and fourth plans increased the involvement of the *panchayat* in the development process, the central government continued to carry most of the responsibilities for transportation, communications, and agricultural development (GoN, 1970; Savada, 1993).
- *Fifth Five-Year Plan (1975–1980)*: It mentioned poverty for the first time although no specific goals were set. Top priority was given to agricultural development, with emphasis placed on increasing food production and cash crops, such as sugar cane and tobacco. Increased industrial production and social services also were targeted, as well as controlling population growth (GoN, 1975; Savada, 1993).
- *Sixth Five-Year Plan (1980–1985)*: Agriculture remained the top priority followed by increased social services, with reduced allocations for transportation and communication since it was deemed more beneficial to increase spending on agriculture and industry (GoN, 1980; Savada, 1993).
- *Seventh Five-Year Plan (1985–1990)*: It encouraged private sector and local government participation in the economy and targeted increased productivity in all sectors, expanding opportunities for productive employment, and fulfilling the minimum basic needs of the people. It set specific goals for the first time relating to the availability of food, clothing, fuel-wood, drinking water, primary healthcare,

sanitation, primary and skill-based education, and minimum rural transport facilities (GoN, 1985; Savada, 1993).

- *Eighth Five-Year Plan (1991–1996)*: Though the political upheavals in the mid-1990s derailed development planning, there was a proliferation of NGOs involvement in development during this period (Fujikura, 2001; GoN, 1991).
- *Ninth Five-Year Plan (1997–2002)*: The goal was to increase economic growth and alleviate poverty and unemployment; NGOs were encouraged to partner with local development organisations, especially in backward communities in underdeveloped and remote regions (GoN, 1997). They worked through district and village development committees, local municipalities, educational institutions, and CBOs (Dhakal, 2007).
- *Tenth Five-Year Plan: Poverty Reduction Strategy Paper (PRSP) (2002–2007)*: With international development policy on the Millennium Development Goals (MDGs) firmly influencing development in Nepal, the PRSP had four pillars: (i) Broad-based economic growth; (ii) social sector development, including human development; (iii) targeted social inclusion to bring the poor and marginalised groups into mainstream development, and targeted programs for ultra-poor, vulnerable, and deprived groups; and (iv) good governance (GoN, 2003; Shrestha et al., 2008). The Local Self-Governance Act (GoN, 1999) aimed to encourage local governance of development, continuing the focus on partnership outlined in the ninth plan (Dhakal, 2007).
- *Interim Three-Year Plan or Eleventh Plan (2007/8–2009/10)*: It continued the focus on inclusive economic growth, poverty alleviation, and employment creation (Shrestha et al., 2008) and meeting the MDGs (GoN, 2008).
- *Three-Year Plan or Twelfth Plan (2010/11–2012/13)*: It reflected an increasing shift toward self-reliance or community responsibility for development as the focus on local participation and governance became further entrenched within the PRSP and MDGs (GoN, 2011c).
- *Three-Year Plan or Thirteenth Plan (2013/14–2015/16)*: It emphasised inclusive and participatory development by encouraging government, non-government, and private organisations to work in coordination to alleviate poverty and increase economic growth (GoN, 2014).

Shrestha et al. (2008) observed,

> Development planning in Nepal started in 1955 with the first five-year plan and subsequently ten five-year plans have been drawn up and implemented. The first four plans emphasized infrastructure development. From the fifth and sixth plans emphasis shifted towards agriculture and industry. Poverty alleviation was the major objective of the seventh, eighth, ninth and tenth plan periods. To alleviate poverty and attain sustainable food security is a challenge for Nepal. It can be achieved by making a shift from subsistence farming to a commercialized and diversified system of agriculture.
>
> (p. 97)

From the end of the first five-year plan (1956–1960) to the seventh (1986–1990), the *Panchayat* system dominated; 'each village was represented by a group of elders in a council or "Panchayat" which formed part of a pyramid of such bodies with the King at its apex' (Crane, 2002, p. 2). As previously discussed, under monarchic rule, Nepal had averred political organisations and banned all political parties. However, political parties operated clandestinely, mainly among the elites of urban Kathmandu and in the Terai Region.

To escape prosecution, many of Nepal's political leaders fled to India and ran clandestine political activities from there. As a substitute, the *Panchayat* system, run by rural elites, comprised six government-sponsored class and professional organisations for peasants, labourers, students, women, former military personnel, and college graduates. These organisations represented group or class, rather than national interests, and offered the only open political forum. Political leaders based in India, who had formed the NCP and the Communist Party of Nepal (the two main political groups), infiltrated these *panchayat* organisations that controlled most of the development projects in the country during this 30-year period (1960–1990). Government-sponsored and controlled development was not only a means of macroeconomic planning but also a way to keep the populace compliant (Dahal, 2002). Most services were government owned and controlled (Shakya, 2012).

However, there were changes afoot that led to the NCP holding its first national convention in 30 years in Kathmandu, which was attended by delegates from all political parties, including a multiparty delegation from India. With the United Left Front parties, a coalition of seven communist factions, the NCP launched the Movement for the Restoration of Democracy to replace the *Panchayat* system with a multiparty political democracy. Thus post-1990, Nepal began to follow neoliberal, post-development policies, privatising services and allowing NGOs to flourish (Fujikura, 2001). International development policy promulgated by the Bretton Wood institutions promoted INGOs, and bilateral and multilateral foreign aid organisations into the state's development apparatus. Hundreds of development projects initiated and funded by the UNDP, the World Bank, the Asian Development Bank (ADB), the United States Agency for International Development (USAID), and numerous INGOs entered the country. Despite international intervention, however, historical powerful elites continued to undermine the movement to democracy being promoted by international development organisations (von Einsiedel et al., 2012a, 2012b; Hutt, 2004; Lawoti, 2012; Lawoti & Pahari, 2010; Panday, 2012). Thapa (2007) explained the sentiment of civil society at the time:

> Yet, if – through the peace process – the extremists to the right and left can be contained in the democratic centre, we might finally be able to establish a democracy that doesn't just look like a democracy, but that acts like one as well, a democracy that embraces the current women's rights and *Dalit* rights movements, and the movement for the rights of ethnic nationalities, the sexual revolution, the movement for local ownership of natural resources, the trade union and labour rights movements . . . we want social and economic equality as well . . . [that] is simply to say that we want democracy.
>
> (p. 260)

However, the country's political leaders lacked the institutional infrastructure and political will to promote democratic arrangements to serve the interests of the people. The group and class elites from the *Panchayat* system did not want to let go of power thus declining living standards, intermittent ethnic conflict, natural disasters, and human rights violations hampered peace and development processes in civil society.

Through this political turmoil, INGOs continued to fund and provide technical support to a broad spectrum of development projects in Nepal concerned *inter alia* with poverty reduction; rural and urban development; healthcare; education; peacekeeping and conflict management; social security for women, children, and youth; forestry, agriculture, and environmental sustainability; and democracy, human rights, social justice, and civil society.

Poverty reduction

O'Connor (2002) believed poverty and development were two sides of the same coin; without poverty, there would be no development and *vice versa*. Yet, despite decades of development in Nepal, poverty persists. Official figures show that 23.8 percent of the Nepali population lives on less than USD1.25 per day (UNDP, 2014b). Nevertheless, INGOs involvement has achieved moderate poverty reduction from 25.2 percent in 2011 to 23.8 percent in 2014. With the influence of the MDGs, a third of the 211 INGOs affiliated to the SWC (SWC, 2015a) were primarily concerned with poverty reduction, though all INGOs worked towards poverty alleviation.

Rural development

Poverty was highest among Nepal's rural population, which constituted 83 percent of the population (UNDP, 2014b). Large families, food insecurity, poor nutrition, a lack of primary healthcare and safe drinking water, overcrowded smallholdings, social discrimination, and high rates of illiteracy were among the major concerns for rural development INGOs (International Fund for Agriculture Development, 2014). Crane (2002) described Nepal as

> a primarily agricultural country, with farm products amounting to 41% of GDP and farming provides 77% of what employment there is. Most of this agriculture is subsistence farming. Land is a very important issue to many Nepalis.
>
> (p. 8)

Nepal's rural population was 'labour-rich' but far from 'land-rich' and 'life-rich'. Shrestha et al. (2008) reported that two-thirds of Nepal's population was engaged in agriculture:

> It is estimated that there are about 40,000 NGOs and 200 INGOs involved in development activities in Nepal. As rural livelihoods are basically dependent on agriculture, most of these NGOs and INGOs are involved in agriculture and rural development activities.
>
> (p. 108)

In 2009, the government embarked on the Project for Agriculture Commercialization and Trade (PACT) within the Ministry of Agriculture Development. The project, which continued until 2018, aimed to improve the competitiveness of smallholder farmers and the agribusiness sector in selected commodity value chains. For the most part, however, rural development and local governance has been beset with problems of collusion and corruption, such that there were no local government elections (The

Asia Foundation, 2012; Gellner & Hachhethu, 2008) in the rural areas between 1997 and 2017. As a report by The Asia Foundation (2012) explained,

> Local-level corruption in Nepal is generally not a onetime event, but rather an ongoing practice involving a multitude of stakeholders each playing their part. In other words, it is not a complete absence of the rule of law in local governance, but rather an ethical degeneracy in local politics that seeks short-term individual benefits at the cost of longer-term public welfare, and deeply undermines formal procedures of governance. Collusive schemes employed at the local level included a tactical mixing of private and public interests in resource allocation decisions, practice of nepotism, lack of transparency, [and] informal decision-making, among others.
>
> (n.p.)

Despite the enactment of the Local Self-Governance Act in 1999, 'difficulties in implementation, particularly due to the capacity crunch at the local level, disjointed planning, and the onset of conflict . . . [rendered it ineffective as] an enabling instrument for local bodies to take control of their affairs' (The Asia Foundation, 2012, n.p.). The report of The Asia Foundation (2012) further noted that, following the expiry of locally elected representatives' tenure in 2002, government-authorised civil servants assumed the functions of the local bodies. Since these government functionaries lacked the capacity and ability to command local legitimacy, they compromised decision-making among local leaders:

> [They] had to rely almost entirely on relationships rather than procedures to perform their duties. By 2009, this coping strategy was adopted as the preferred political framework and acquired formal legitimacy with the formation of All Party Mechanisms (APMs) . . . [in which] no party is uniquely positioned to monopolize public funds and resources for patronage purposes.
>
> (The Asia Foundation, 2012, n.p.)

Thus, evolved the culture of local governance 'in the context of conflict and transition, and in some ways as reverberations of historical problems in Nepali society, politics and the state' (The Asia Foundation, 2012, n.p.). Against this backdrop, NGOs and INGOs filled the rural development vacuum through integrated and participatory rural development approaches to improve the quality of rural lives. Some INGOs working in rural development are shown in Table 3.2.

Urban development

Due to the harsh conditions of rural poverty, people flocked to urban centres in search of sustainable livelihoods. A lack of industrialisation and economic development had led to the country's status as one of the least urbanised nations in the world, with only 6.3 percent of the population living in urban areas in 1981 rising to 8 percent in the early 1990s. At the time, only 23 settlements were designated as urban areas, and only the capital city of Kathmandu had a population above 100,000. With Patan (also called Lalitpur) and Bhadgaon (also called Bhaktapur), the Kathmandu Valley in the Hill Region had the largest concentration of the total urban population (almost

Table 3.2 Rural development INGOs

INGOs	Activities	District covered	Beneficiaries
AMDA-MINDS	Integrated maternal and child health, empowering women's group for nutrition and reproductive health, infectious disease control, particularly malaria, HIV and AIDS, and TB, improving access to basic health services, and capacity building of health volunteers	2	
Blueberry Hill Charitable Trust	SAFAL (Sustainable Access to Finance and Livelihoods in Nepal) – financial services to low-income households, and micro enterprises (60% of recipients are women)	6	28,000
Child Fund	Education, community development	2	3,850
Foundation Nepal	Community development (health and sanitation, education, and community mobilisation) and participation of *Dalit* and disadvantaged groups	1	11,010
Good Neighbours International Nepal	Education, health, water, and sanitation, family livelihood improvement, community partnership	13	26,830
Habitat	Environment, advocacy, and emergency relief		
Helvetas	Agriculture, community development, economic, and business development, environment, and forestry	75	812,628
Tearfund	Integrated community development incorporating health, livelihoods, education, and child at risk work	3	12,500
Finnish Evangelical Lutheran Mission (FELM)	Education, food security, health, and sanitation, community development and peacebuilding, child mental health, and disability	30	213,405
ISIS Foundation	Holistic community development in Humla, child protection and development, and child repatriation	2	10,000

Source: Adapted from AIN (2014)

40 percent). Fourteen of the 23 settlements were located in eastern and central Terai. There were no urban settlements in the Mountain Region (Savada, 1991). Not only was Nepal predominantly rural, but also the existing urban settlements were neither well-developed nor well-connected in terms of their geographical distribution, with the only real urban network in the central quadrangle comprising Kathmandu, Pokhara, Butawal, and Hetauda.

With an annual urban growth rate of 4.7 percent, by 2011, 17 percent of Nepal's population had gravitated to its 58 urban centres (GoN, 2012b). This brought numerous problems for urban planners, ill-prepared to cope with this influx of people

(Tibaijuko, 2007). Politically, the decade-long Maoist insurgency contributed to this dramatic increase in the urban population as the rural population fled unrest (Crane, 2002; von Einsiedel et al., 2012a, 2012b; Hutt, 2004; Lawoti, 2012; Lawoti & Pahari, 2010; Panday, 2012).

The urban areas were only marginally better (Devkota, 2012). Unplanned development had left them chaotic, polluted, and overcrowded with an increasing belt of slums and informal settlements. Socioeconomic and sociospatial inequalities had engendered violence, conflict, and crisis, while the increasing privatisation of public services and housing was occurring alongside decreasing public assistance and social security. Cognisant of the lack of management and urban planning from negligent authorities (Devkota, 2012), INGOs introduced initiatives to improve urban livelihoods (see Table 3.3).

Healthcare

Nepal's progress on the MDGs was driven by the Tenth Five-Year Plan and Poverty Reduction Strategy Paper (2002–2007) (GoN, 2003), as well as the Interim Three-Year Plan (2007/8–2009/10) (GoN, 2008). By 2011, the infant mortality rate had declined from 108 in 1990 to 46, and the under-five child mortality rate from 162 to 54 per 1000 live births (GoN & UN Nepal, 2013). With a per capita income of USD712, life expectancy at birth was 69.1 years (UNDP, 2013). However, the 2013 joint GoN and UN report claimed this progress would not be sustainable unless health stakeholders continued to improve health provision for deprived and disadvantaged communities.

Nepal's complex geography presents major challenges to health services in remote villages, where traditional practices, service inaccessibility, and a lack of transportation exist. Increasing marketisation, a fragile health insurance system, neglected health policies, and a lack of political commitment further reduces the accessibility and affordability of healthcare in Nepal. As the World Health Organisation's Commission on Social Determinants of Health (2008) noted, the unequal distribution of health inequalities is 'not a "natural" phenomenon but is the result of a toxic combination of poor social

Table 3.3 Urban development INGOs

INGOs	Activities	Districts covered	Beneficiaries
Care	Women and girl's empowerment, sexual reproductive health, emergency preparedness and disaster risk management, migration and urbanisation, food security and climate change, and gender-based violence	39	1,816,432
Practical Action	Disaster risk reduction, maximising benefits from basic services, sustainable urban environment, healthy home and clean air action, water sanitation and waste management amid the growing urbanisation, and cross-cutting areas, such as climate change and making markets work for poor	20	64,347

Source: Adapted from AIN (2014)

Table 3.4 Health INGOs

INGOs	Activities	District covered	Beneficiaries
Action Contre La Faim	Nutrition, mental health and care practices, food security, water, sanitation, hygiene, and emergency	1	3,816
The Britain Nepal Medical Trust	Promoting quality health services and ensuring health rights	45	75,000
Centre for International Studies and Cooperation	Community health	60	70,000
Cetro Cooperazione Sviluppo Onlus	Quality education and health	5	10,000
Centre for Reproductive Rights	Reproductive health rights	3	
Micronutrient Initiative	Health and nutrition	26	566,000
Netherlands Leprosy Relief	Health and disability	25	8,981
World Vision	Maternal child health, nutrition, water sanitation, and hygiene	11	279,485
Marie Stopes Nepal	Reproductive health and family planning	30	200,000
CBM Nepal	Eye health, ear health, physical disability, mental health, inclusive education and community-based care	35	393,432

Source: Adapted from AIN (2014)

policies and programs, unfair economic arrangement, and bad politics' (p. 1). INGOs working to promote affordable healthcare in Nepal are shown in Table 3.4.

Education

Survival in the knowledge economy relies on a strong education system, which, in turn, depends on high literacy rates. Development in most areas focuses on the acquisition of knowledge, skills, and competencies in, for example, HIV and AIDS prevention, women's reproductive health, gender inequities, and teenage pregnancy. Education is essential to a strong socioeconomic order and is valued, too, for its transformative potential as a force for liberation and democratisation (Maclure, Sabbah, & Lavan, 2009). Though committed to free and compulsory primary education, the government lacked the capacity to implement its policies and deliver quality educational programs. Thus, 'a comprehensive, integrated humanitarian approach, including food aid, nutritional support and economic aid to families, is needed to help . . . children' (Integrated Regional Information Networks [IRIN], 2010, n.p.) missing out on education.

In Nepal, 39.1 percent of citizens in the age group of six were illiterate (GoN, 2011a), though there were low-literacy areas in two-thirds of the country (IRIN, 2010). Large numbers of children were deprived of their basic right to education (IRIN, 2010; GoN & UN Nepal, 2013). The United Nations International Children Emergency Fund

(UNICEF) (2015) reported that the 2015 earthquake exacerbated this worsened condition of the children that left a million children out of school. It was also concerned that

> great strides made over the last 25 years in increasing primary school enrolment in Nepal – from 64 per cent in 1990 to more than 95 per cent today – could suffer a serious setback in the aftermath of the earthquake. Nepal's high dropout rate was already a major concern. Around 1.2 million Nepali children between the ages of five and 16 have either never attended school or have dropped out.
>
> (UNICEF, 2015, n.p.)

This added to the consistent disparities in access to education across geographical areas and social groups (IRIN, 2010). The challenge to keep children in school arose from the combined impact of poverty, HIV and AIDS, disabilities, early marriage, and the exploitation and trafficking of children (GoN & UN Nepal, 2013). IRIN (2010) reported that, while Nepal has 7.3 million students in the school system at the primary, secondary, and high school levels:

> There are more than 100 ethnic groups in Nepal, half of which are indigenous and regarded as marginalized, while 22 are classified as 'extremely disadvantaged'. They make up about 40 percent of the country's 29.3 million inhabitants, while almost one-third of . . . Nepalese live below the poverty line on less than US$1 a day. These groups also have the lowest number of children in schools. . . . They all come from the most exploited communities who are impoverished, suffer from social inequalities and most children have dropped out of school to work in risky situations.
>
> (n.p.)

The government of Nepal has yet to address issues relating to broader socioeconomic qualities, ethnic discrimination, and the exploitation of children, and, more narrowly the quality of, infrastructure for, and general learning environment for children in school. Political instability and low economic growth have impacted on literacy levels, and on the development of access roads to schools located far from students' home villages. Several INGOs collaborate with government to enhance the quality of education in Nepal through funding scholarships, educational programs, training educators, and building infrastructure (see Table 3.5).

Peacebuilding and conflict management

Nepal's long history of political and ethnic conflict, deep-rooted ethnic discrimination, deepening socioeconomic inequalities, and the Maoist insurgency has seen the advent of peacebuilding and humanitarian INGOs that operate in post-conflict situation (Bhattachan, 2000; von Einsiedel et al., 2012a). As Collier, Elliott, Hegre, Reynal-Querol, and Sambanis (2003) observed, with prolonged conflict comes a persistent 'legacy of poverty and misery' (p. 20). Nikolov (2009) noted,

> Nepal underwent internal armed conflict during 1996–2006, and today many [international and local] NGOs are actively engaged in Nepal to build peace, support development and human rights, and to aid the democratization process.
>
> (p. 1)

Table 3.5 Education INGOs

INGOs	Activities	District covered	Beneficiaries
Asia Onlus	Education	3	10,000
Educate The Children	Education	2	1,850
Intervita Onlus	Children's education	2	
Room to Read	Literacy and gender equality in education	12	154,732
Rural Education and Development	Education, enterprise, social development and information communication technology through community library	39	1.86m
Strømme Foundation	Quality education – formal and non-formal, literacy, and life-skills training	7	25,000
World Education	Formal, non-formal, vocational, and health education: It has supported more than 150,000 children by rescuing them from exploitative work conditions, providing scholarships and helping parents find income-generating activities	22	473,500

Source: Adapted from AIN (2014)

Table 3.6 Peacebuilding INGOs

INGOs	Activities	Districts covered	Beneficiaries
Mennonite Central Committee Nepal	Peacebuilding	12	20,000
Saferworld	Building sustainable peace Gender and security People-centred local safety Conflict sensitivity Reducing armed violence and conflict Capacity building Research	7	9,000
The Asia Foundation	Conflict transformation and peacebuilding	70	

Source: Adapted from AIN (2014)

INGOs make an enormous contribution to peacekeeping and conflict management through their programs and activities (see Table 3.6).

Social security for women, children, and youth

Due to the legacy of the traditional feudal patriarchal system and the state's lack of commitment to implementing its existing gender-related policies, women, children, and young people are highly vulnerable groups in Nepal. Women constitute 51.5 percent of the population, children 39 percent, and young people 19.38 percent (GoN, 2011b). Yet, national policy has long ignored issues relating to the socioeconomic and educational status of women, children, and young people in Nepali society.

Nepal's gender inequality index is extremely low at just 0.479 and 28 percent of married women experience physical and/or sexual violence (GoN & UN Nepal, 2013; UNDP, 2014a). Early marriage is common with 40.7 percent of children marrying by the age of 18 years and almost 4.7 percent of school-age children not enrolled in school (GoN & UN Nepal, 2013; UNICEF, 2013). IRIN (2010) reported,

> More than one million children in Nepal work as domestic servants, porters, carpet weavers, bricklayers and miners . . . there are about 55,000 children working as domestic servants and more than 16,000 in adult establishments, such as massage parlours and dance restaurants.
>
> (n.p.)

The International Labour Organization (2013) reported that only 2.7 percent of population were in paid employment and 90 percent of the economically active population were involved in the informal economy. Unemployment is extremely high with few opportunities for young people in the country.

The government is heavily dependent on the support of international, multilateral, and bilateral organisations to improve the quality of lives of women, children, and youth in Nepal. INGOs are instrumental in *inter alia* funding and conducting grassroots programs, and improving the technical competencies of local NGOs and CBOs to improve the well-being of women, children, and youth (see Table 3.7).

Forestry, agriculture, and environmental sustainability

Agriculture is the backbone of Nepali society. It employs 70 percent of the population and contributes to 33 percent of the GDP (UNDP, 2014b). Reductions in arable land have led to food insecurity and increasing reliance on imported foodstuffs, as the existing agriculture sector is unable to fulfil the demand of a growing population (New Spotlight, 2014). Likewise, once known as *hariyo ban Nepal ko dhan* (greener forest; Nepal's wealth), forests have shrivelled from 4.8 million to 3.6 million hectares in last 20 years (Food and Agriculture Organization of the United Nations, 2010). Nepal is the fourth most vulnerable nation in the world to climate change and lost USD170 million to natural disasters in 2014 alone (UNDP, 2014b).

Ten percent of Nepal's landmass comprises dangerous glacial lakes and an average of two deaths per day is due to disasters making it highly vulnerable to environment risks (UNDP, 2014b). Many INGOs conduct awareness among local people about agricultural subsistence, sustainable forests, and environmental conservation (see Table 3.8).

Democracy, human rights, social justice, and civil society

Although Nepal's first experience of democracy was in 1951, the country still struggles to democratise its institutions rooted in authoritarian, elitist practices (Cedric, 2009; Crane, 2002). As explained earlier, not only is the Nepali population fragmented by caste, ethnicity, geography, and economics, it is also linguistically diverse. Though its

Table 3.7 Women, children, and youths INGOs

INGOs	Activities	Districts covered	Beneficiaries
Women			
Fondazione Un Raggio di Luce Onlus	Women's empowerment, livelihood support, and microfinance	3	5,238
Heiger International Nepal	Women's empowerment benefitting families	27	57,135
Stichting Veldwerk the Netherlands	Women's development	4	14,000
Children			
Associazione Amici Dei Bambini	Children's development	11	25,000
Child Protection Centres and Service International	Child protection	16	10,000
Save the Children	Child rights and child protection	66	1,976,368
Terre des hommes Foundation	Child protection	4	19,230
Shangrila Home VZW	Underprivileged children's development	1	200
World Mobilization	Child protection and anti-trafficking	6	3,000
Youths			
Mercy Corps	Youth engagement	21	
PlaNet Finance	Microfinance, youth employment, business development	4	600
Search for Common Ground	Youth and peacebuilding	15	
Winrock International	Youth entrepreneurship and development	33	430,080

Source: Adapted from AIN (2014)

many ethnic groups each have distinct traditions, dress, and languages, in general terms, Crane (2002) reported,

> They divide into those of Mongolian origin in the high areas of the West and East and those of Indian origin in the Valley, lowlands and the Terai. Nepali is the lingua-franca. Tribal groups can be ordered by caste: Gurungs, Magar, Rai, and Limbu form, for example, a middle, agricultural caste. Newars and Chettris tend to be of higher caste along with Brahmins, with Sunars and Khamis being examples of lower, artisan caste. Though caste is less important in Nepal than India, it is possible to generalize that the higher castes are at the center of the intellectual and political elite of the country. Middle and lower castes are under-represented.
>
> (p. 7)

Table 3.8 Agriculture, forestry, and environmental INGOs

INGOs	Activities	Districts covered	Beneficiaries
Agriculture			
Lutheran World Relief	Agriculture and food security	3	3,083
Norlha-Helping People in the Himalayas	Agriculture and food security	3	895
USC Canada Asia	Agriculture and natural resource management	8	35,000
Environment			
Deutsche Management Akademie Niedersachsen	Environment and climate change	10	
Red Panda Network	Biodiversity, climate change, environment, and sustainable development	3	79,997
Forestry			
Mountain Institute	Conservation of mountain environment and preservation of mountain culture	5	30,545

Source: Adapted from AIN (2014)

Historically, CHHE have dominated national politics and there is a great deal of discrimination against low-caste people (O'Donnell, Cullel, & Iazzetta, 2004). As Lawoti (2012) explained,

> Dalit, indigenous nationalities, Madheshis, and Muslims were particularly discriminated against and repressed. [The state's] . . . tight control and effective oppression largely succeeded in surpassing public resistance, resulting in deceptive façade of peace and ethnic harmony, which the state tirelessly propagated through school textbooks, an official narrative of Nepal's history, and the media. It was a 'peace' based on hierarchy and inequality among groups and maintained through coercive force.
>
> (p. 129)

Social inclusion is not high on the agenda as Nepal continues to straddle the authoritarian-democratic divide (Freedom House, 2015) and political elites continue to dominate its post-republic 'partocracy' more concerned with power than institutionalising democracy (Michels, 1915).

At the inception of Nepal's experience with multiparty democracy, Shah (1993) argued it required additional motifs to become a nation; it needed to institutionalise democracy in a manner that would include its diverse ethnic and cultural groups, which, has yet to be accomplished. Several INGOs work closely with the Nepali government to manage its democratic transition, support its evolving public administration, and institutionalise the rule of law to create better conditions for democracy, human rights, and social justice (see Table 3.9).

Table 3.9 Democracy, good governance, and human rights INGOs

INGOs	Activities	Districts covered	Beneficiaries
BBC Media Action	Works to improve dialogue and debate between the public and those in power in Nepal. Issues covered include maternal and child health and political accountability, strengthening resilience in response to climate change. Its ground-breaking TV and radio debate program *Sajha Sawal* (Common Questions) reaches a national audience of 6.5 million. Its innovative improvised radio drama *Katha Mitho Sarangiko* raised public awareness on social and health issues, such as maternal and child health and gender-based violence	75	6.5m
Pact Inc	Builds empowered communities, effective governments, and responsible private institutions. Focuses on local governance, HIV and AIDs, livelihoods, natural resource management, and peacebuilding	6	6,053
Demo Finland	Good governance and democracy	14	10,000
DanChurchAid	Reaches households educating them on inclusive citizenship for accountable governance	14	40,000

Source: Adapted from AIN (2014)

AIN (2014) claimed that INGOs shared significant portion of the total foreign aid budget through their development activities and, also, employ over 4000 Nepali citizens in the country. Despite their significant contribution, people are divided on whether INGOs are 'saviours' in Nepal's failing development or 'creative destructors' generating widespread dependency and preventing the government from being fully accountable to its diverse peoples.

INGO culpability for failed development

Critics see foreign aid as a sleeping pill, helping people cope rather than dealing with their sleeplessness. INGOs, in a sense, reinforce government inertia and let government off the hook by filling in the gaps for its inefficiencies. Some believe Nepal has overdosed on development aid. Although Nepal's development planning started in 1955 (Shrestha et al., 2008), by the advent of democracy in the golden decade of the 1990s, it had already been pronounced a failure (Bista, 1991; Karan & Ishii, 1994; Khadka, 1991; Panday, 1999; Shrestha, 1997) due *inter alia* to its complex geography, the legacies of exploitative rulers, and the ineffective implementation of 13 successive development plans. Some of the blame was laid at the door of INGOs that spoon-fed corrupt politicians and bureaucrats (Bell, 2014).

Solutions were seen to lie in the participation of local people in development planning, with INGOs playing a major role in this (Karan & Ishii, 1994). Dependency theorists blamed foreign aid organisations for obstructing progress (Bista, 1991) and called for reduced reliance on external intervention (Khadka, 1991). Panday (1999) argued that failed development was not necessarily due to inadequate inputs into development, but rather to the lack of vision of people in power and their inability to shape development institutions, enforce appropriate development frameworks, and promote value systems in keeping with national and local social realities. He saw foreign donors and INGOs as complicit in this state of affairs (Panday, 1999, 2012).

Shrestha (1997) saw the borrowed concept of Western development as itself problematic and out of step with Nepali social realities. From his neo-Marxist perspective, he saw the propagation of Western development models in Nepal as designed to position foreign donors and INGOs as superior to the Nepali population. His analysis also encompassed indigenist and decolonised sentiments to the extent that he described the arrival of Western development as instrumental in colonising the minds and bodies of Nepal's diverse peoples. To him, foreign aid and international organisations had produced nothing but a 'trail of victims' in Nepal.

British-born journalist Bell (2014), in his account of the history of foreign aid and development in Nepal, pronounced it an unmitigated failure noting aid programs had failed to help poor people. Nepal's failed development can be traced across three stages, 'from the forbidden kingdom to the blank slate', 'becoming a pet country', and 'rentier state', to which might be added the Millennium Development Goals and human development.

From forbidden kingdom to blank slate

Until 1951, Nepal remained a mystery to most foreigners as the then rulers restricted outsiders fearing they would enlighten their citizens and undermine their power. Edmund Hillary's conquest of Everest in 1953 with Tenzing Norgay Sherpa brought Nepal to international attention. At about this time, Nepal was inaugurated as a development laboratory through US-style community development, which was subsequently adopted by Indian, Chinese, and Russian development experts bent on modernising Nepal. These outsiders considered Nepal a blank slate as Nepali society was oblivious to the external world (Bell, 2014). Once Nepal joined the UN in 1955 and agreed to the Colombo Plan in 1956, the UK, Switzerland, Norway, and Japan emerged as new custodians of Nepali development. Poverty reduction became the mantra of development actors from the 1960s to1980s through economic growth and basic needs approaches. Importantly, these nations also brought their non-government organisations along with them. These became significant actors in the later period of Nepali development.

Becoming a pet country

In 1990, the regime changed from an absolute monarchy to a multiparty democracy. The then King Birendra accepted the idea of a new constitution inspired by liberal Western democracy, including universal suffrage, a two-tier government, independent judiciary, and the right to equality and freedom for all. In the wake of its fledgling democracy, Nepal became international donors' 'pet country' (Bell, 2014) as aid started to flow into the country. The World Bank and the International Monetary Fund pushed Structural Adjustment Programs to create growth through their privatisation and liberalisation agendas, which benefited a few elites, while rural growth did not materialise. During this period, the idea of partnership and sector support opened doors for many European donors and INGOs that still influence Nepali development policies and programs. However, the state of underdevelopment did not radically reverse, despite the aggressively pursuits of international donors and non-profit aid agencies. Dixit (1997) noted,

> The powerful aid-givers, all strong believers in the trickle-down theory, are of the belief that when the dust settles the public as whole will benefit. More likely we will have a revolt on our hands, but by then of course the aid agencies will be on to the fad of the next . . . [several] decades – which will in all probability be, and not at all incongruously, the rediscovery of the role of government in national development.
>
> (p. 183)

Rentier state

At this point, Nepal became a 'rentier state', Mahdavy's (1970) term widely adopted in political science and international relations theory for states which derive all, or a substantial portion of, their national revenues from the rent of indigenous resources to external clients. This theory sees development as creating dependency.

Human development and the Millennium Development Goals

Nepal was successful not only in bringing down the Maoists, but also in regime change from a monarchy to a republic. This raised people's expectations for radical growth and accelerated progress, though the promised constitution, which has yet to find its way through the broader consciousness of all political parties. Nepal embraced the inclusive, participatory, people-centred human development approach and Millennium Development Goals in 2000s. Though narratives of development and development jargon echo through government offices, donor discourse, and INGO seminars, the fruits of Nepali development, like a walnut, are locked inside and Nepal remains an example of failed development to this day. In a lengthy manner, Bell (2014) opined,

> Political protection is accorded to orphanages that traffic children, and the licensing of sub-standard medical schools. The transport sector is controlled by transport syndicates, tripling the price of road haulage and killing but passengers. The syndicates insist that their drivers are exempt from the traffic laws . . . food wholesale is controlled by fruit and vegetable cartels, driving down farmers' income and generating food-price inflation. Union bosses create a monopoly on factory workers, then use it to enrich themselves, crippling industry against the interests of workers. Fuel is distributed . . . by fuel cartels, which shut off supply when their interests are threatened; drinking water is supplied by drinking-water cartels because the water board is dysfunctional . . . goldsmiths have a syndicate [who reject testing quality of gold and their scales]. Taxi cartels defend the right to rig metres. [Even] construction companies have contractors' cartel, which build the country's substandard

infrastructure at inflated costs, from the development budget. [In other words, Nepal has no place for rule of law and systematic development agenda causing poor to become poorer and rich to richer].

(pp. 338–339)

Panday (2011), too, questioned Nepal's 60 years of stagnant development and poverty, and demanded accountability from donors:

> Much of the malaise is the result of ineffectual Nepali institutions and actions. . . . However, given the symmetrical relationship between foreign [and INGO] aid and development in Nepal and the embedded unequal donor recipient relationship, foreign aid [and INGO involvement] cannot escape scrutiny and responsibility for what has not happened.

(p. 11)

Panday (2012) claimed Nepal's failed development was due not only to political failure but also to sociocultural and institutional factors. Though INGOs and foreign aid added significantly to people's empowerment, social mobilisation, and service delivery, 'critical development failures can be attributed at least in part to donor [and INGO] fatigue or reluctance to invest in productive sectors that could generate broad-based economic growth with equity and justice' (Panday, 2012, p. 94).

In summary, INGOs seemingly have compounded Nepal's failed development as they provide fertile ground for Nepali authorities to move away from their responsibilities. If INGOs truly want Nepal to reverse the curse of failed development, then they need to revisit their roles in designing and implementing development policies and strategies. In the event of failures of governance, INGOs must challenge Nepal's development authorities by stopping or at least curtailing future disbursements instead of increasing aid and program volumes. Only then will INGOs become true partners in development (Panday, 2012).

Costs of development

The criticism against INGOs is not that they contributed nothing to Nepal's development, but that they have done so at great cost. On the face of six decades of engagement, billions of dollars spent, and hundreds and thousands of pieces of expert advice provided, what INGOs have helped Nepal achieve is unsatisfactory in Bell's (2014) opinion. INGOs have sponsored every aspect of development, as shown in the range of areas in which they are engaged (as discussed above). Yet, Nepal is far from building a strong institutional foundation for social justice and a redistributive economy for sustainable future development, growth, and democracy. Rather than address political issues and structural change, INGOs have romanticised the development domain. This has led to development forays into Nepal being described as 'Adventures in Aidland' (Mosse, 2011) and a 'leaf in a begging bowl' (Vikala, 2000). Many believe that INGOs have their own hidden agendas that have nothing to do with the national interest. A frequent criticism is that they do nothing about the deep-rooted social and cultural discrimination, government inaction, and political power plays. As evidence shows, the Maoist insurgency was due, not only to the uprising of Maoist leaders and ineffective government policies but also to the effects of poverty, inequality, and political and ethno-linguistic division in the country with which INGOs failed to engage (Fujikura, 2001; Hutt, 2004; Lawoti & Pahari, 2010).

INGOs import development buzz words from global trends discussed in conferences by think tanks based in New York, Vienna, Bern, and Paris that have nothing to do with Nepal and the discriminatory, patriarchal, hierarchical practices that obstruct poor people's access to development (Bonio & Donini, 2009). Panday (2012) believed various actors', including INGOs', selective amnesia was, and continues to be the critical issue to the government's failure to integrate Nepal's multicultural and multilingual sociocultural structure into national politics. But Nepal is in a double bind, dependent on INGOs that generate aid and employment and sponsor a large share of the country's financial, technical, ideological, and human resource development, when they also play a role in generating conflict and breeding corruption with their focus on the supply side of development cooperation (Panday, 2011) and productive economic growth (Uvin, 1998). Panday (2012) notes INGOs have not had a significant effect on agriculture, though most of the population lives on subsistence agriculture, while the industrial sector has never been a recipient of INGO funding (Shakya, 2012). The tendency of INGOs to work through a chain of intermediaries rather than 'give directly to the poor' (Hanlon, Barrientos, & Hulme, 2010) is seen as a breeding ground for corruption in the country.

Patronage and politicised bureaucracy are the major impediments to Nepali public services. The political parties and their leaders misuse insecure and ambitious bureaucrats, who then easily engage in illegal overtures for personal gain (Panday, 2012). The INGO penchant for pouring excessive aid into the country provides a safe passage for lawmakers and bureaucrats to dodge their legal accountabilities. INGOs exacerbate this situation by channelling monetary, technical, and human resources to a corrupt government:

> Corruption is a fundamental systemic issue [in Nepal]. . . . In terms of political economy, we provide the fiscal space for . . . [corrupt officials and politicians] to do what they want to do. The donors [including INGOs] do not want to speak openly because each one is into 'let's give peace a chance'.
>
> (Bell, 2014, pp. 343–344)

INGOs in Nepal have become equated with sustaining and strengthen ruling elites (Mishra, 2007). Dixit (1997) believed this delivered nothing but chaotic and lopsided progress:

> [It] has centralized power and privileges in Kathmandu valley. It has pampered the old money, and has also helped to create and intoxicate Nepal noveau riche from the central secretariat to the village roundtable – as represented in government's inability to mobilize domestic resources . . . as well as the loss of cooperative spirit among villagers. Whereas earlier, the rural peasantry would come together to build a suspension bridge or maintain Chautara (trail rest), the overwhelming tendency now is to wait for the 'project appraisal team' of a government, INGOs and NGOs.
>
> (pp. 177–178)

Importantly, Shrestha (1997) and Pigg's (1993) indigenist and decolonised lenses make INGOs outcasts in Nepal's traditional and collective societies. Shrestha (1997) argued that foreign-assisted humanitarian activities cloaked in exploitative capitalism intended not only to colonise Nepali peoples but also to buy support for the policies of donor countries and development agencies. Pigg (1992, 1993), a social anthropologist, argues the alternative to development must be sought from Nepali social interaction and movements that operate outside of imported and dominant development discourses. She not only challenged the existing development models propagated through international humanitarian aid agencies but also demanded they revisit the very idea of development while working in Nepal. She argued imported development strategies have constructed a space that regulated and controlled human behaviour. Rather localised development needed to bring lived experiences into focus and give people ownership of development programs. Nepali development actors needed to challenge the ambiguous image that foreign development actors had constructed of Nepal and the Nepali village (Pigg, 1992).

Shrestha (2000) believed that foreign aid agencies and INGO support for development in Nepal was more like an 'open class war ranging . . . across the landscape, from urban trenches to rural fringes' (p. 154). The peculiarity of this war is that it involves no soldiers, no arms, and no blood, but a very powerful colonial and imperial tool of modern history – development. Like a Shakespearean tale of mischief and misery, these development initiatives are, for Shrestha (2000), maddening and sickening. They have intoxicated and trapped Nepali peoples with their money and rhetoric. They offer hope for 'haves-nots', while leaving the 'haves' – the controlling class – in power. The relationship between INGOs and Nepali authorities might be seen as a walnut – the shell of the walnut (international agencies) admits no localisation of their intervention strategies, while the inner kernel (Nepali authorities) sheds no light on changing current stagnation. Thus, the international agencies and government authorities employ reciprocal strategies to exonerate one another. The failure of international aid or humanitarian agencies in the country is like an open secret. Brusset and Regmi (2002) claimed aid had sustained Kathmandu's elite patronage system:

> Society's caste employment and income inequalities are indeed strikingly reflected in many [local and international non-government development] agency structures . . . [despite] the emphasis given to rural employment, the management of programmes is still overwhelmingly placed in the hands of a gatekeeper group [such as few elite and expats].
>
> (p. 15)

Likewise, the European Union Conflict Assessment Mission openly acknowledged that civil society or local NGOs through which donors and INGOs spent tens and hundreds of billion were 'a very small group of English speaking elite operating in Kathmandu' (Van Lookcke & Philipson, 2002, p. 21). Kumar (2000) noted that only 15 percent of Nepali people benefited from foreign aid and most were either powerful bureaucrats or leading business people. The media, which are considered the fourth organ of the state, refrain from reporting these issues since they derive a hefty income from advertising for INGOs and government agencies (Bell, 2014). Activists and professionals too, like social workers, are in a double bind, dependent on INGOs for employment thus forgoing activism to sustain their livelihoods.

Conclusion

Nakhau bhane din bharko shikar; khau bhane kanchha bauko anuhar – a popular adage among Nepali people – provides an apt description of INGOs in Nepal. It literally represents a hunter's dilemma. After his hunt had yielded a monkey at the end of the day, the hunter asks himself, should I eat or starve? INGOs portray a similar dilemma. Nepal cannot refrain from INGO-led development, as it does not have the capacity to address development issues and it must do this knowing that INGOs will likely never equip Nepali people to become fully self-supporting (Fujikura, 2001; Shrestha, 1997, 2000).

This chapter has outlined Nepal's dependency on foreign aid and the important role played by INGOs in providing humanitarian assistance and development support. This is another context alongside Nepali society from which the concept of decolonised and developmental Nepali social work has emerged. As outlined in the following chapters, since there are no formal jobs for social workers within the state and civil society apparatus, most graduates of Nepal's mushrooming social work education programs are finding employment in INGOs operating in Nepal's capital city of Kathmandu. This is taking them into the domain of social development when their education equips them for US-style social work within a welfare infrastructure that does not exist within Nepal. The next chapter will outline the context of social work education in Nepal.

Chapter 4

Social work education in Nepal
A brief historical perspective

In this chapter I examine the history of social work education in Nepal, a recent development that has yet to be granted government legitimacy and widespread community sanction. I begin with a discussion of the key chronological milestones in the development of higher education, the establishment of Tribhuvan University (TU) in 1959, the first National Education Plan in 1971, the entry of private sector provision in 1980, the National Education Commission in 1992, and recent developments post-2013. I, then, turn to the development of social work education from its colonial roots to its rapid growth, followed by a period of disillusionment with an absence of formal positions for social work graduates. Thereafter, I also examine contemporary developments relating to the structure of social work education programs and major issues in social work education, and end with a brief discussion on the future of social work education and practice.

In the last 22 years, social work education in Nepal has expanded from one university to four and almost 50 affiliated colleges. As outlined in Chapter 2 and Chapter 3, Nepal has long been influenced by Westernisation and academic institutions have followed the path of imported knowledge and embraced foreign concepts since the introduction of social work education in 1996, which persists even today. As discussed earlier in Chapter 1, social work in Nepal is built on knowledge borrowed from the USA, filtered through Indian influences. Nepali social work education, therefore, draws heavily on the work of Western scholars and uses mainly US textbooks and theories. Hence, imported knowledge from the USA and, to a lesser extent, Europe has come to be considered essential and there has been little attempt to decolonise or contextualise social work education and practice to enhance its relevance to local Nepali people.

Social work has become a global profession with a strong commitment to culturally sensitive and anti-oppressive practice to promote locally relevant practice. However, there are several forms of oppression, especially by developed nations in the Global North over developing countries in the Global South. Hence, social work education and practice in Nepal is not free from external influence and this creates tension for those seeking to develop decolonised social work (Gray, Coates, Yellow Bird, & Hetherington, 2013b; Jenlink, 2004; Khinduka, 2007; Martinez-Brawley & Zorita, 1998).

Historical development of higher education in Nepal

The history of higher education in Nepal spans less than a century. Until the beginning of the 20th century there were no efforts by any parties – public, private or public and private partnerships – to develop a higher education system in this small Himalayan nation. The development of higher education went through several stages: (i) The early period (1918–1956); (ii) the establishment of the first university (1959); (iii) the development of a national education plan (1971–1976); (iv) the advent of private sector provision (1980); (v) the education commissions of 1983 and 1992; and (vi) the recent developments in higher education system (post-1993).

Early period (1918–1956)

Tri Chandra College was the first institution of higher education in Nepal established in 1918. Founded by Chandra Shamsher Jang Bahadur Rana, this college was started in affiliation with Calcutta and then Patna University in India. It later became affiliated to TU, the first institution of higher education in Nepal, established in 1959. This institution brought hope for many Nepali citizens, since it provided affordable education in their home country. However, located in Kathmandu, it was not accessible to all Nepali people. In 1929, the Ayurbedic School at Naradevi, again in Kathmandu, was established for training in medicine. There followed training in forestry (Department of Forestry) (1947), law (Nepal Law College) (1954), education (College of Education) (1956), and nursing (Nurses Training School) (1956) in Kathmandu. The Nepal National College opened in 1956 (Regmi, 1997).

Establishment of TU (1959)

Established in 1959, TU is the backbone of higher education in the country. Prior to this time, most students had to go to universities in India or elsewhere. Not only did it provide opportunities for students to study in their home country, it also provided for the redesign of higher education curricula, previously dominated by Indian universities (Centre for Economic Development and Administration, 2007).

National Education Plan (1971–1976)

The National Education Plan (1971–1976) was product of the Nepal Education Planning Commission (1954) and Nepal All-Round National Education Committee (1961). Its aim was to produce human resources with scientific and technical education for development. It sought to counteract the elitist bias of the inherited system of education by linking it more effectively to Nepali productive enterprises and egalitarian principles (GoN, 1971). Also, the National Education Plan aimed to bring academic and organisational change in the field of education (Centre for Economic Development and Administration, 2007).

Private sector provision (1980)

By 1980, there was heavy growth in student enrolment for higher education in the country and TU alone could not accommodate entire student population. Hence it started affiliations with private colleges nationwide. By 2013, there were more than 702 private colleges affiliated to several universities in the country (University Grant Commission [UGC], 2011). From their inception, these private colleges generated controversy about whether they were service- or market-driven.

National Education Commission (1983 and 1992)

In 1983, the Government appointed a Royal Commission on Higher Education, which launched the Nepal Sanskrit University (NSU) in 1986. In 1992, the National Education Commission was appointed to review the education system. The Commission recommended the need for a UGC, the decentralisation of education, and the establishment of regional universities. Notably, the Commission led to the establishment of Kathmandu University (KU) (1992), Purwanchal University (PU) (1994), and Pokhara University (PoKU) (1997).

Recent developments in higher education in Nepal (post-1993)

Higher education in Nepal has grown in importance in recent years. The government's efforts to establish the Bisheshwor Prasad Koirala Institute of Health Science, with the support of the government of India, in 1993; Lumbini Bauddha University (LBU) in 2005; and Mid-Western University (MWU) and Far-Western University (FWU) in 2010 were milestones in the ongoing development of Nepal's higher education sector. In addition, the government established the Agriculture and Forestry University (AFU) in 2010 in Rampur, Chitwan in the central part of the country. There has been a huge expansion of colleges and universities, higher education enrolment, number of students, academics, and graduates, as shown in Table 4.1, providing increased access to education in the country. Nevertheless, significant numbers of students continue to migrate to foreign countries for higher education.

Development of social work education in Nepal

As mentioned earlier in Chapter 2, Nepal has witnessed numerous social, economic, political, and cultural crises since unification. The recent turbulence following the Maoist insurgency has left the entire Nepali society in transition. The lack of clear direction has left people feeling frustrated and hopeless about the future. The decade of 1990s was important for many reasons. In 1990, Nepal shifted from an absolute monarchy to a constitutional monarchy and a multiparty democratic system was established. In 1996, the Maoist insurgency sought to eliminate feudalism and bureaucratic capitalism (Bhurtel & Ali, n.d.). This was when social work as an academic discipline was introduced in the country. Since 1996, its development has passed through several phases.

Beginning phase: colonial root of social work education (1987–2004)

In 1987, Brother James F. Gates launched Social Work Training at the SWI. In 1993, Father William Robins, then president of the Jesuit Society of Nepal, joined him. The SWI initiated a training program for government and NGO workers. The SWI was heavily influenced by US social work methods grounded in medical and psychological perspectives. It became independent in 2001, when it was formally registered with Nepal's SWC. It runs nine-month social work training programs in Kathmandu (SWI, 2013).

US Jesuit missionary Father Charles Law initiated bachelor degree in social work at St Xavier's College, an affiliate of KU, in 1996. The people of Nepal remained oblivious to this new discipline and it was unclear how it fit the national level's (Pawar & Tsui,

Table 4.1 Higher education institutions in Nepal

Universities and academies and date of establishment**	Number of higher education campuses				Students, academics, and gradates			
	Constituent campuses	Community campuses	Private campuses	Total campuses	Female %	Students Total	Teachers Total	Graduates Total
Universities n = 9								
TU, 1959	56	296	526	878	42.5	353718	*13679	58109
NSU, 1986	6	1	10	17	15.5	1798	770	478
KU, 1991	6	0	15	21	42.5	9658	341	1572
PU, 1994	4	0	49	53	32.6	16666	116	1053
PokU, 1997	3	5	106	114	39.5	24726	49	3924
LBU, 2005	1	0	0	1	3.0	33	NA	NA
MWU, 2010					Newly established universities			
FWU, 2010								
AFU, 2010								
Academies with university status n = 3								
B. P. Koirala Institute of Health Sciences (BPKIHS), 1993	1	0	0	1	41.4	1072	183	246
National Academy of Medical Sciences (NAMS), 2002	1	0	0	1	46.3	203	142	NA
Patan Academy of Health Science (PAHS), 2009	1	0	0	1	30.0	60	85	NA
Total	83	302	702	1087	41.8	407934	15365	65382

*Includes community campus academics
**Excludes foreign-affiliated university campuses (n=32)

Source: Adapted from UGC (2011)

2012) integrated development plan. However, it set in train an Indian strain of US social work education, which had little to do with sociopolitical events in the country at the time – the transition to a multiparty democracy and the Maoist insurgency resulting from endemic and persistent poverty, wealth inequalities, regional disparities, and the chronic failure of governance at the centre (Bhurtel & Ali, n.d.), as shown in Figure 4.1.

Rather than respond to the needs, welfare, and rights of people suffering the worst economic, social, and political injustices, from the outset, social work education was grounded in the US medical and psychiatric model at a time when medical and psychiatric assistance was not a priority. The nation needed human power with social work skills and knowledge to respond to poverty and inequality and the emerging crisis arising from the Maoist insurgency in 1996 (Nikku, 2010b). Its US missionary progenitors set in train a form of social work with a colonising mission, which has proved extremely resistant to engaging with the sociopolitical, cultural, and economic realities of life for most people in the country.

In 1997, TU instituted Social Services as a subject at the Bachelor of Arts (BA) level at its Padma Kanya Multiple Campus for female students in Kathmandu. The brainchild of Dr Padma Lal Devkota, a professor of sociology, this course was later renamed a BA in Social Work in 2005. The BA in Social Work is taught in most of the private

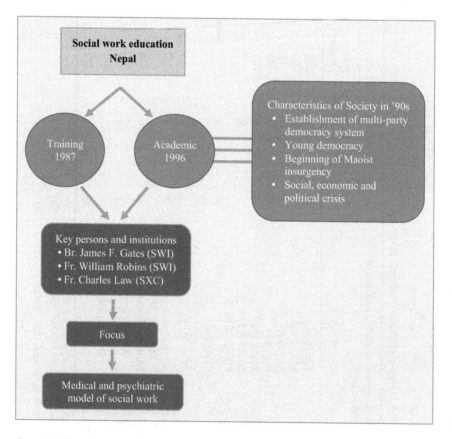

Figure 4.1 Development of social work education in Nepal

colleges in Kathmandu due to TU's liberal approach to affiliation. The first BA in Social Work at Padma Kanya College was not as popular as St Xavier's program, which was taught largely by social work educators from the USA and India. This situation persists even today. St Xavier's served as the role model for social work education. It continues to promulgate an Indian-influenced Western model of clinical social work, which is incompatible with the Nepali cultural milieu and remains unresponsive to widespread sociostructural problems and inequalities in Nepal (Nikku, 2010b, 2014).

Popularisation phase: attraction towards social work education (2005–2010)

Until 2005, very few people in the nation knew about social work education. Most of its students were drawn to a career in not-for-profit NGOs and INGOs in Kathmandu. Its popularity took hold when K and K College and the Classic International College launched its course in 2005. Both courses were taught by part-time social work graduates, who provided lectures and field supervision but had little to do with course planning and implementation beyond this. Sujeet Karna and Manoj Sah, alumni from Nirmala Niketan in Mumbai and Delhi School of Social Work in New Delhi, were among the first to teach social work in those colleges, which remains dominated by sociologists and other non-social work professionals.

In 2005, PU instituted a BSW and MSW in its affiliated Kadambari Memorial College of Science and Management and St Xavier's College, respectively. Two Indian academics, Dr Bala Raju Nikku and Mr Joyson Jose, are credited with initiating social work in PU that offered social work education in its affiliated colleges located in Kathmandu. Both served as Head of the Department of Social Work at St Xavier's College. With several non-social work Nepali scholars including Pranita Bhushan Udas, Pradipta Kadambari, the late Komal Magrati, and Promod Dhungana, social work education took root at PU. Dr Bala Raju Nikku, and Professor M.N. Mishra, a retired professor of Public Administration, led the further development of social work at PU (Nikku, 2013).

Given the high demand for these courses, other institutions began offering social work education but there was no proper vision and direction to its development. Also, none of these colleges is bound to regulatory educational standards or a professional code of ethics. To date, there has not been any monitoring and evaluation from relevant bodies, such as the UGC or Ministry of Education.

Nevertheless, Kadambari Memorial College of Science and Management has attempted to popularise social work by celebrating World Social Work Day for the first time in 2008, given its founders' association with the international and regional social work organisations. Social work academics in Kathmandu have created the false impression that social work is a legitimate, community-sanctioned profession in Nepal, when, in truth, little is known beyond the universities in the nation's capital (Nikku, 2010b). With most social workers, who have managed to find employment, working in externally funded NGOs and INGOs in Kathmandu, social work has yet to reach the grassroots. This has led to criticisms of it being an elitist profession.

Period of disillusionment: questioning the legitimacy and direction of social work (2011 onwards)

There is growing dissatisfaction among social work graduates in Nepal. First, since the government has not developed policies to embed social work in the social fabric, there is no legitimation of graduates within the central administration. Second, the citizenry is unaware of the social work profession. Thus, social workers lack community sanction (Nikku, 2010b). Ideally, an institutional approach is needed, whereby social work is shaped to cater for the entire nation, with the 125 ethnic groups falling within its sphere of influence. A localised Nepali model of social work would address social injustice and indigenous disadvantage, and promote community strengths. Nevertheless, despite the absence of institutional and community legitimation, social work education continues to grow with MWU having introduced a BSW and MSW in 2012, TU an MSW in 2015, and FWU preparing for an MSW.

Contemporary scenario of social work education in Nepal

Social work education continues to attract students beyond the Kathmandu valley, with many young people from different parts of Nepal aspiring to become professional social workers and contribute to social development. In any country, the aim of social work education should be to meet the needs of people in society (Chang & Mo, 2007). However, a clear agenda for the future development of social work education in Nepal needs to examine the composition and structure of programs on offer in universities and colleges to assess their relevance to the needs, problems, and issues of Nepali society.

Structure of social work programs

Social work education in Nepal includes three tiers:

- Social Work Training.
- Bachelor of Social Work.
- Master of Social Work.

Social Work Training

The target of Social Work Training programs is employees of government and non-government organisations attempting to enhance their social delivery by learning the basic concepts and skills of social work. The SWI offers social work training to produce trained community animators and service facilitators (SWI, 2013).

Bachelor of Social Work

The Bachelor of Social work varies across universities. KU and MWU offer a four-year generalist BSW. TU and PU offer a full-time, three-year BSW with a focus on social services and rights-based social work, respectively.

Master of Social Work

MWU and TU provide a full-time MSW on a semester basis that include a fieldwork component. The MSW offered by TU is an extended form of its BSW. MWU only offers MSW program with specialisation courses in community development, rights-based social work practice, and social organisation and human resource management.

Curriculum content

The three main universities – KU, PU, and MWU – offer compulsory courses in social casework, social groupwork, social welfare administration, social action, community organisation, social work research, sociology, human behaviour, social policy and legislation, and development communication within their BSW and MSW programs. KU also offers a compulsory course in computer education. However, course contents vary greatly across the four universities – TU, KU, PU, and MWU – and 50 colleges, teaching social work.

Fieldwork

Fieldwork is an integral part of social work education but there is insufficient consultation between social work educators and public and private agencies on curriculum development. Also, fieldwork requirements vary. PU and KU have a compulsory fieldwork requirement of 24 and 16 hours a week, respectively, while TU requires its students to complete 250 hours of fieldwork a year. Only MWU has a written syllabus for fieldwork, with precise guidelines specifying the respective roles and responsibilities of students and field supervisors. The MWU fieldwork course includes communication skills, rapport building, recording, and ethical decision-making.

Influence of international organisations on social work education

International exchange was commonplace given the ease of communication through information technology. Social work professionals around the world believed in the professional development and internationalisation of social work education (Greif, 2004; Nimmagadda & Martell, 2008; Strug, 2006). International social work organisations – IASSW and IFSW, and their regional affiliates, such as APASWE in the Asia-Pacific region – worked continuously to increase the global reach of the profession. Kadambari Memorial College of Science and Management and Thames International College, affiliates of PU and TU respectively, had joined international social work organisations to enhance the exchange of communication on the development of social work and assume a controlling and leading position to direct social work in Nepal. Social work graduates have attempted to develop a strong link between the international and regional social work bodies and Nepali social workers. These ventures into internationalisation and globalisation have not, however, benefited the development of culturally relevant social work education and practice in Nepal.

Major issues in social work education

After two decades, social work education and practice in Nepal faces many challenges (Kharel, 2013; Nikku, 2013) relating to curriculum content, pedagogical methods, fieldwork placements, social work's legitimacy, privatisation of social work education, the future direction of social work, and the development of culturally appropriate theory and practice. Students have complained about out-dated curricula, pedagogical methods, and the poor teaching skills of social work educators, many of whom are not social work trained. The wider adoption of a critically reflective approach will enhance cultural relevance. Finally, most graduates are unable to get jobs in social work once they have completed their social work degrees and lack motivation to pursue higher degrees to enhance educational and practice standards (Kharel, 2013).

Fieldwork education requires improvement, while the profession lacks systems, guidelines, and a code of ethics to guide practice. Furthermore, since most agency supervisors are not social work trained and come from diverse disciplines, there is a disjunction between university-based education and fieldwork practice, with students forced to assume volunteer status in fieldwork agencies (Nikku, 2013).

The social work profession in Nepal lacks official recognition and legitimacy. Nepali social workers' inability to form a united professional body (the one in existence did not represent all social workers in the country) hampers attempts to legitimise the profession. Local communities, along with the SWC and government bureaucracy, have yet to sanction social work as a professional occupation. There is no systematic program to achieve institutional recognition for social work in Nepal or well-planned objectives to shape and guide professional social work. Without strategic direction, social work education will continue to grow and produce graduates rather than competent professional social work practitioners.

The privatisation of education in Nepal means most of the colleges have launched social work education as a profit-generating venture rather than to develop the profession or contribute to the holistic, self-determined social development of the country (Kharel, 2013; Loomis, 2000). Boards or trustees, most of whom have little understanding of social work education and practice, run private institutions.

Hence reform of all aspects of social work education is required, including pedagogical methods, quality of teaching staff, culturally relevant curricula, and professional leadership. Finally, research is needed to ensure social work education and practice are evidence-based and accord with national development organisations and standards, while addressing the needs of local people considering geographical and cultural diversities of Nepal.

Conclusion

Having explored the colonial and imperial roots of social work education in Nepal, the chapter examined the contemporary situation in the country and international influences on the development of its social work education programs. It examined several concerns, not least the lack of culturally appropriate knowledge and curriculum content, an issue much debated in the literature on decolonising social work, discussed in Chapter 5.

Chapter 5

From an imported model to a decolonisation of social work

In this chapter I review the literature on decolonisation in social work. Though a nascent area of social work scholarship, many of its proponents are inspired by egalitarian ideas and solidarity with marginalised and oppressed Indigenous Peoples. Decolonisation seeks not only the reclamation of culture but also political sovereignty for Indigenous Peoples. The chapter begins by examining the nature of imported social work in Nepal before discussing how mainstream social work's universalising mission took place through technology transfer from the West to the rest. Thereafter, it explores and synthesises the growing literature on indigenous social work with the emergent discourse on the need for a shift from imported model to a decolonisation in social work.

Revisiting imported social work in Nepal

As mentioned in Chapter 2, Nepal is often characterised as a *Shangri-La* and is valued for its significantly important geostrategic position in the Himalayas between two emerging nations, India and China. Its tumultuous history, marked by sudden and frequent violent political changes has disadvantaged large sections of the population, especially rural people, who constitute 70 percent of the population and are dependent on subsistence agricultural (Bartlett, Bharati, Pant, Hosterman, & McCornick, 2010). Not only disadvantaged by caste, gender, geographic, and regional disparities, they are also subject to the vagaries of weather and climate and are most likely to bear the brunt of natural disasters and climactic events. In recent years, poverty, unemployment, and declining natural resources have crippled the day-to-day lives of the rural peoples (Thieme et al., 2005). Denied the rights stipulated within national and international human rights conventions (National Human Rights Commission of Nepal & Office of the High Commisoner for Human Rights in Nepal, Nepal, 2011), there are few social protections for most of Nepal's population.

In response, Nepal has imported Western models of social work with a questionable fit with the scenario outlined earlier. Like other nations in the Global South, Nepal struggles to popularise the profession at the grassroots levels. Further, these imported models based on human rights require a representative democracy to support them. Nepal's democracy is tenuous, at best, and its deep caste and ethnic divisions, have little regard for the rights of those at the lower end of the sociopolitical spectrum. This brand of social work has spawned numerous social work education programs, as discussed in Chapter 4, without a rights-grounded context of human service practice. The situation is ripe for the decolonisation of social work, which, despite its hundred-year history in numerous nations in the Global South, struggles to gain legitimacy. Having bypassed the cultures and ethnicities of Indigenous Peoples, the social work profession in the Global South, including India, which has had a major influence on Nepal, has not been accorded the same status as it has achieved in the Global North (Midgley, 1981, 2008). Arguably, the universalisation of social work has not been good for the countries in the Global South, which views it as vehicle of imperialism and colonialism (Gray & Coates, 2008; Gray & Hetherington, 2013; Yunong & Xiong, 2008; Ling, 2004; Midgley, 1981; Nimmagadda & Balgopal, 2000; Osei-Hwedie, 2002; Strug, 2006; Weaver, 1999; Yan & Tsui, 2007). Midgley (1981), a key scholar on professional imperialism, argued,

> Social work formulated in the nineteenth century reflected prevailing Euro-
> pean and North American cultural values and political ideologies. Individualism,
> humanitarianism, liberalism, the work ethic and capitalism unrestricted by govern-
> ment intervention were regarded as virtues by founders of social work in the West.
>
> (p. xii)

These founders in the USA were Mary Richmond and Jane Adams, who differed on social work as a scientific profession (Brieland, 1990; Lundblad, 1995; Pumphrey, 1956). Adams favoured a path of community-based cultural and urban reform, by voluntary workers, that even today best approximates the community development ethos perpetuated by national governments and international development agencies in the Global South (Lundblad, 1995; Midgley, 1981).

Modernising social work

As already outlined, as an instrument of universalising modernisation, social work seeks to spread its Western ideals of liberalism, democracy, and social reform. Its organisations work to transform social work into a global profession grounded in these universal values through their regional networks. Payne (2005) argues that social work is modernist because

> it is based on the idea that we can understand and study social problems and soci-
> eties, and take rational action to deal with the problems we see. . . we can reach a
> rational understanding of human beings and society and decide how to act con-
> sistently to change both people and societies according to our knowledge. Having
> a theory that guides action is inherently modernist – it says that we can base our
> actions on evidence of the world around us.
>
> (pp. 15–16)

Modernising social work runs aground in the Global South because 'the evidence of the world around us' on which it is based comes from a context far removed from where it is being transplanted. For the Global South, it is non-indigenous knowledge, being imposed in a colonising and imperialistic way, because it overrides and ignores local cultures and ways of life, and is not suited to the kinds of problems requiring solution. To plug the gap, various bodies of knowledge have developed, as Gray, Coates, Yellow Bird, and Hetherington (2013b) note,

> As an emerging field within the discipline, Indigenous social work draws on a num-
> ber of multiple, often conflicting and competing discourses, including indigenization;

cross-cultural practices, culturally sensitive social work practice, cultural appropriateness, cultural competence and cultural safety; anti-oppressive, anti-discriminatory
and anti-racist practice; international social work; decolonization theory; Indigenist research and Indigenous standpointism; social ecology or environmental
(green or eco) social work; and spirituality. . . . Questions surrounding who has
the right to speak for whom; whether there is a place for non-Indigenous social
workers in Indigenous social work; and the ethics of conducting research with
Indigenous communities strike at the heart of these oftentimes polarizing debates.

(p. 14)

Ironically, these bodies of knowledge have Western origins, but indigenous scholars
draw on, and seek to develop, indigenous, culturally appropriate theories and models
that are more sensitive to indigenous, that is, non-Western, ways of knowing and
being. Decolonisation scholars have furthered this knowledge-development process
by going beyond cultural appropriateness to further the political agenda of indigenous
and marginalised peoples, the *Janajatis* and ethnic minorities in Nepal. Like indigenous social work, decolonisation is concerned with the rights of Indigenous Peoples,
political processes that incorporate historical and cultural priorities; recognise imperialistic vested interests; take account of ethnocentric differences; recognise Indigenous
Peoples' rights to land, language, and spirituality; and continue the long-standing
struggle against hegemonic forms of practice (Gray et al., 2013b, 2013c; Gray & Hetherington, 2013; Midgley, 1981, 2008; Rao, 2013). Decolonising social work draws
on many sources, including the sociology of globalisation (Giulianotti & Robertson,
2009; Gray & Hetherington, 2013). It explores and debates on homogenising processes, expressed in terms like Americanisation, Westernisation, modernisation, and
McDonaldisation, as a counterpoint to heterogenising processes, expressed in terms
like localisation, contextualisation, and 'Nepalisation'. The latter represent and draw
insider perspectives to counter the Othering that goes on in the professional discourses
seeking internationalisation and universalisation. In other words, decolonisation seeks
to counter the modernising thrust of development and professional social work that
arises from outside in the Global North. It resists external standards that destroy local
social networks and cultural practices and disempower local communities. It also resists
internal networks and cultural practices that disadvantage social groups, for example,
cultural norms and practices that disadvantage those at the bottom of the caste, ethnicity, and religion hierarchy (Rao, 2013). What unites indigenous and decolonisation
scholars is the desire to challenge those who claim that we are living in a post-colonial
era. As Briskman (2008) notes, while colonialism might have formally left the nations
of the Global South, its legacy remains wherever external agencies seek to dominate
the lives of local peoples. Both indigenous and decolonisation seek self-determination
and sovereignty (Ives & Loft, 2013; Mokuau & Mataira, 2013) and bring people
together for solidary progress.

Technology transfer: from the West to the rest

Many models of technology transfer have been advanced. In the social work literature,
there are three region-specific models (Cox, 1995; Ragab, 1995; Resnick, 1995). Cox
(1995) examined the transformation of social work in the Asia-Pacific Region and its
evolution from pre-colonial traditional practices to missionary philanthropy and charity
and colonial welfare administrations. The philanthropic charity model evolved into the

voluntary or non-government sector that worked in tandem with the colonial government welfare system. These colonial institutions focused mainly on urban problems and sought to professionalise the welfare system by training welfare personnel in Western social work models, despite local resistance.

Ragab (1995) documented the process of social work diffusion into the Middle East and Egypt. Its first phase was rapid transformation as US models of social work training were imported into Egypt between 1935 and the 1960s. Starting in the early 1960s, strong dissatisfaction with this US model of social work and the subsequent Islamisation of social work marked the beginning of authentic social work in Arab countries.

Resnick (1995) traced the development of social work education in South America, where it followed a similar colonial path on its way from Europe and the USA beginning in 1925. Social work gradually became indigenised as the profession became shaped by South American cultures, and social and political realities. By the mid-1960, localised social work was accepted as important to social development in South America.

Mayadas and Elliot (1997) highlighted the global development of international social work in the 20th century. The early pioneers expanded social work in Europe and the USA between the 1880s and 1940s. The second phase of professional imperialism followed in the era of colonialism between the 1940s and 1970s, when social work spread to Africa, Asia, and South America. The third and fourth phases of reconceptualisation and indigenisation between 1970s and 1990s led to regionalisation and localisation in international social work and social development.

An analysis on these models reveals that the roots of social work in the Global South are not indigenous and locally driven. The profession spread from the West with local academics and practitioners questioning its fit with non-Western contexts from the outset (Gray, Coates, & Yellow Bird, 2008b; Nagpaul, 1972, 1993; Nimmagadda & Balgopal, 2000; Osei-Hwedie, 2002; Walton & Nasr, 1988; Yunong & Xiong, 2008), including Nepal (Gray & Yadav, 2015; Yadav, 2016).

An account of technology transfer would be incomplete without an examination of the way this transmission of Western knowledge was possible and why it proliferated rapidly around the globe, especially in the Global South. This technology transfer was driven by the supremacy of the English language, modernising development and professionalising missions by wealthy, powerful Western agencies and universities, the inability to indigenous scholars to devise a locally relevant academic curriculum, and the lack of publications in the vernacular on indigenous contexts and practices (Coates, Gray, & Hetherington, 2006; Gray, Coates, & Yellow Bird, 2008a; Nimmagadda & Balgopal, 2000).

English is the lingua franca for social work education around the globe, since North American and British universities established most of the social work departments across the world (Haug, 2005). Today, most social workers are trained in, or encouraged to, learn English to further international social work. Also, Western academics and practitioners, who are economically privileged and can travel around the world to attend conferences and seminars, and run projects portray their concepts, methods, and techniques as superior to local ones (Coates et al., 2006). In addition, Coates et al. (2006) noted,

> This technology transfer occurred with the support of the United Nations and international humanitarian organizations despite the recognized 'need to promote

indigenous methods, curricula and study material'. . . . 'Thus, even among IFSW member countries, often a majority of social workers are excluded due to lack of professional qualification'. . . . When there is such an imbalance of power, exchange is almost impossible to achieve.

(p. 383)

Nimmagadda and Balgopal (2000) elaborated the concept of 'West is best' in relation to their experience from India. They noted, 'The notion that anything from the West is the best was the dominating characteristic of the first phase of technology transfer and indigenization' (p. 8). Third World nations or Global South adapted Western activities while critical of the 'West is best' approach because of its awkwardness of fit in indigenous communities. They advanced a dialogical model of technology transfer, a two-way model of knowledge translation, with mutual learning characterising knowledge development (Nimmagadda & Martell, 2008).

The IASSW and IFSW promote technology transfer through their international and regional conferences and meetings. Social workers from the Global South support the efforts of these organisations and build alliance at international, regional, and national levels. However, they do not necessarily promote the interests of Indigenous People and, in the past, have been damaging to the knowledge of Indigenous Peoples in the Global South.

Indigenous social work: concept and construct

Criteriology is a neoscholastic term referring to the science of criteria, or concepts building knowledge constructs, such as indigenous social work. Theory development in indigenous social work draws on the work of Western and non-Western scholars. Hetherington (2009) provided a comprehensive theoretical framework on indigenous social work (see Table 5.1). She included indigenisation, cross-cultural practice, critical perspectives, and eco-spiritual approaches, all of which were Western perspectives, to construct culturally situated social work, which she described as 'elusive, open-ended, emerging, and flexible but rooted in culture' (Hetherington, 2009, p. 17). She raised several questions about indigenous social work:

- What defines indigenous social work?
- Is it defined by the ethnicity of the person or their practice style?
- Is Western-style casework indigenous social work when it is carried out by indigenous social workers?
- What defines indigenous social work practice?

(Hetherington, 2009)

Midgley (2008), too, questioned whether indigenous social work was limited to First Nations Indigenous People and their cultures and whether it, too, was an imperialist hegemony (rooted as it was in standpointism). Indigenous scholars are sceptical about the indigenisation discourse, since it weakens First Peoples' political agenda, leading Gray et al. (2008a) to wonder whether it was an outmoded concept. They identified parallel discourses on indigenous social work, one emanating in the literature on indigenisation in Africa, Asia, and South America, and the other in scholarship on Indigenous First Nations social work in Australia, Canada, and the USA.

Table 5.1 Analytical framework for literature review

Literature	Associated terms	Theoretical influences
Indigenisation (older literature)	• Authentisation • Professional imperialism • Technology transfer	• Enlightenment thinking • Modernist • Developmental, that is, indigenisation sees development as progress
Cross-cultural practice	• Culturally sensitive • Culturally appropriateness • Cultural competence • Cultural awareness • Cultural safety • International social work	• Multiculturalism • Globalisation
Critical perspective	• Anti-oppressive practice • Indigenist, standpointism • Political • Decolonisation • Anticolonial and post-colonial • Whiteness	• Critical, radical, Marxist, and feminist • Post-modern and social constructionist • Structural and post-structural • Ethnicity and cultural studies
Eco-spiritual perspective	• Holism • Connectedness • Ecosystems	• Systems and ecosystems • Ecology and spirituality • Phenomenology • Narrative (oral storytelling)
Culturally situated Indigenous social work	• Culturally relevant • Culturally embedded	• Hybridity • Critiques of cultural • History • Discourse analysis • Research into 'natural helping'

Source: Hetherington (2009, p. 17)

Historical roots of indigenisation in the Global South

The debate on indigenisation and authentisation in social work seemed to originate with Shawky's (1972) seminal paper in Egypt. But, cultural analysis is almost as old as the history of professional social work itself especially initiated by Adams (1902) in *Democracy and Social Ethics* and Richmond (1907) in *Good Neighbours in the Modern City.* Post-war Third Worldism, however, triggered the indigenisation movement (Boroujerdi, 2002) spurred on by the deep realisation among people in the Third World of being systematically alienated by the Western world (Atal, 1981).

The fifth international survey of social work training found strong resistance to US social work theories (Walton & Nasr, 1988). Shawky (1972) was one of the first to write about the lack of fit between imported social work and local contexts, calling for a process of indigenisation. Resnick (1995), working at the Catholic University of Chile, likewise, found similarities in the South American experience. She defined indigenisation as 'the process of relating social work functions and education to the cultural, economic, political and social realities of a particular country' (Resnick, 1976, p. 22). As Ferguson (2005) later reported, here indigenisation came from 'local values and concepts including liberation theology, dependency theory, subjective and objective realities, solidarity, conscientisation, praxis and critical theory' (p. 521). Indigenisation led Egyptian social workers to view indigenised social work in the Middle East as Islamic social work (Ragab, 1995, 2017).

The dramatic rise of social work in China revivified the indigenisation debate in social work (Chan & Chan, 2005; Cheung & Liu, 2004; Li, Han, & Huang, 2012; Tsang & Yan, 2001; Wong, 2002; Yan & Cheung, 2006; Yan & Tsui, 2007; Yip, 2005a; Yunong & Xiong, 2008). In China, indigenisation is a combination of Chinese collectivist cultures, values, norms, and spirituality (Confucianism).

In India, indigenisation led to the embrace of Gandhi, Ambedkar, and other social reformers' ideas (Rao, 2013) as social workers sought to deal structural issues, such as patriarchy, casteism, ageism, and the hegemony of Hindu culture and tradition (Alphonse, George, & Moffatt, 2008; Kulkarni, 1993; Mukundarao, 1969; Nagpaul, 1993; Nanavathy, 1993; Nimmagadda & Balgopal, 2000; Nimmagadda & Chakradhar, 2006). Despite ongoing attempts to indigenise social work in India, it remains an unfinished project, due to the durability of Western ties (Rao, 2012).

Al-Krenawi and Graham (2008) observed the economic, emotional, and social ties in Bedouin communities in Israel, where the problem of individuals was the problem of the entire family. This led them to conclude indigenisation as the integration of communal, collective, and familial perspectives in social work (Al-Krenawi & Graham, 2008). They preferred the term localisation as it provided 'insights into social work location, to outline how social work nonetheless can use case vignettes as a modestly useful tool in localization efforts and to integrate spirituality as a useful means for localizing social work' (p. 153).

Graham, Al-Krenawi, and Zaidi (2007) observed that, from the very beginning, social work training in Pakistan was tailored to the cultural and social environment, where 'good social work must be without any external support, it must be indigenous, which can be solved internally and having no competition in it' (p. 631). The foundation of indigenous social work was 'community trust', which was only possible by respecting populations' cultures and traditions. Yunong and Xiong (2008) believed indigenisation involved building an indigenous foundation, such as a philosophical base, theories, working principles, and developing strategies and approaches to address local social problems drawing on local community expertise.

Reactions to technology transfer

Many scholars have criticised social work's impact on the Global South (Al-Krenawi & Graham, 2001; Ferguson, 2005; Gray, Yellow Bird, & Coates, 2008; Ling, 2003, 2004; Midgley, 1981, 2008; Nimmagadda & Balgopal, 2000; Rao, 2012; Walton & Nasr, 1988). Gray et al. (2008a, pp. 11–15, 2008b, p. xiv) used terms like 'McDonaldisation', 'bourgeois model', 'war machine', and 'territorialising agenda' to describe the imperialist nature of social work. They argued that 'McDonaldisation' symbolised a 'one size fits all approach'. Borrowing from Deleuze, Gray and Coates (2008) reference to social work as a 'war machine' is probably one of the most critical depictions of social work, which may not be accepted by all within this field, yet it is true in relation to Nepal.

The IFSW and IASSW maintain their supremacy and authority by rejecting indigenous or cultural minorities' way of helping and healing. Their 'territorialising agenda' is seen in their standardising mission, promulgating an international definition of social work and global standards for social work education. Through their universalising mission, they 'have just over 400 member schools in 55 countries and an estimated 80 member associations around the world representing 500,000 professional social workers' (Gray et al., 2008b, p. xxv). The IFSW (2017) claims its reach has been extended to member associations in 105 countries. In part, this growth reflects the spread of social work in an inclusive Europe, with 37 member associations in 35 countries, and 170,000 social workers now part of IFSW's European Region.

In the early 1980s, Midgley (1981) cautioned social work about its professional imperialism. Advocates of indigenous social work have expressed similar sentiments (Al-Krenawi & Graham, 1996; de Urrutia Barroso & Strug, 2013; Chan & Chan, 2005; Coates et al., 2006; Gray et al., 2008a, 2013b; Hodge & Nadir, 2008; Yunong & Xiong, 2008; Johnston-Goodstar, 2013; Ling, 2004; Nimmagadda & Balgopal, 2000; Nimmagadda & Chakradhar, 2006; Osei-Hwedie, 2002; Ragab, 1982; Rao, 2013; Walton & Nasr, 1988; Weaver, 1999). Almost after three decades, Midgley (2008) observed a 'New Imperialism', in the rise of unipolar international relations dominated by the USA. Social work creates tensions for people in the Global South torn between using professional knowledge and models that seem to have little relevance with situations they are trying to confront, and the requirements of local government administrations far removed from the sophisticated services in the Global North. A closer analysis of the indigenisation discourse revealed several responses to Western social work (see Figure 5.1).

Radical and critical responses: Rejectionist Global South

Critical theorists question the relevance of Western social work as a product of individualism and rationalism, professional imperialism, and colonialism (Drucker, 1993; Midgley, 1981; Nagpaul, 1993; Mukundarao, 1969). They are critical of the impact of Western knowledge, ideology, and technology on non-white countries (Greetz, 1983; Jinchao, 1995; Mohan, 1993). Others see indigenous approaches in the Global South as a form of resistance against imperialistic Western social work (Gray et al., 2008a; Midgley, 1981; Osei-Hwedie, 1993). Thus, indigenisation is a political process seeking self-determination for local, indigenous populations, who have the right to define problems and solutions (Osei-Hwedie, 2002). Atal (1981) identified political and intellectual motivations as the initial drive for indigenisation in Asia, which involved teaching in the national language and use of local materials, as well as research by insiders, who determined research priorities, and theoretical and methodological orientations. Chang (2005) believed indigenisation could take many forms, including attacking the blind adoption of Western concepts and theories to emphasise native studies from an emic perspective. Through theoretical reasoning and grounded research, that is, extensive and careful fieldwork, sociocultural factors can be studied to develop localised philosophies and agendas relevant to indigenous societies.

Osei-Hwedie and Rankopo (2008) discussed the processes and outcomes of developing a social work curriculum at the University of Botswana appropriate to the local sociocultural context. In their opinion, 'social workers could spend their time more productively developing localised knowledge, skills, theories, principles and problem

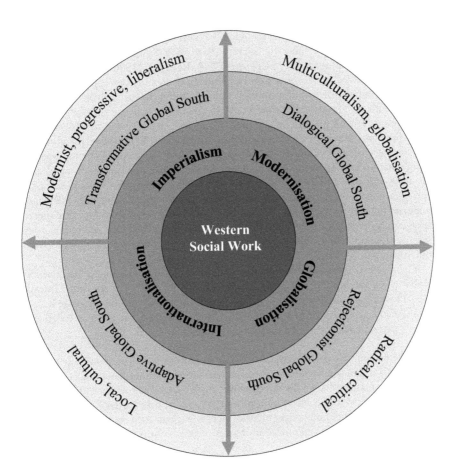

Figure 5.1 Response to Western social work in the Global South

solving strategies relevant to African cultures, world views and ways of life' (p. 217). They believed that 'culturally relevant social work is good social work' (Osei-Hwedie & Rankopo, 2008, p. 217), and indigenisation should 'start from within' as local cultures and helping practices were primary knowledge sources for culturally appropriate social work (Osei-Hwedie, 1993).

While writing about indigenisation and culturally relevant social work practice in Africa, Osei-Hwedie (1996) provided a useful framework of indigenous social work practice, which included worldview; how culture is translated into action; what kind of world/life is strived for; what knowledge is necessary to social work to make a meaningful contribution to people's lives; and what is role of social work practice. He advised to execute indigenous social work practice based upon core determinant composed of social reality, culture, knowledge, institutionalised practice, and education for practice.

Multiculturalism and globalisation responses: Dialogical Global South

This approach acknowledges possibilities in the transfer of knowledge between contexts through dialogical approaches (de Urrutia Barroso & Strug, 2013; Nimmagadda & Balgopal, 2000; Nimmagadda & Cowger, 1999). Bernstein (1996) proposed that indigenisation involved the construction of pedagogical discourse by appropriating other discourse through selective transmission and acquisition to bring them into a special relation with one another. In other words, the result was a hybrid form of knowledge to make social work practice locally specific and context-based and to understand and solve problems from within. Nimmagadda and Martell (2008) called for a two-way knowledge transfer. Nimmagadda and Balgopal (2000) conceptualised six aspects of indigenisation in relation to India: (i) West is best – an inappropriate framework, which produces cultural tensions; (ii) awareness of context – emphasises local needs, issues, and strategies to make social work fit within societal frame of reference; (iii) cultural construction of practice – sees Western social work as a cultural product that alienates Indigenous People; (iv) learning by doing – using local knowledge and popular community development praxis; (v) reflexivity – reflecting on positionality, process, and outcomes; and (vi) thread of creativity – applying imagination to our work.

Yip's (2005a) dynamic model captures the interplay between traditional Asian and global (modern American) culture in the two-way transfer of social work from the global to the local levels and vice versa. Noting the increased cultural exchange between local Asian and modern American global culture, Yip (2005a) suggests to redefine the cross-culture social work as dynamic process in which

> clients' individual subjective and objective profiles and their significant others all have a significant impact on their internalization and interpretation of this vigorous cultural exchange. In the dynamic model, cross-cultural social work is interpreted as a vigorous interaction process among the four parties – workers, clients' significant other and social policy services – in a cultural context consisting of the exchange of Asian and global modern American culture.
>
> (p. 601)

Modernist, progressive, and liberal responses: Transformative Global South

This approach is reformist in nature, as scholars attempt to transform Western social work to match their social, cultural, and political context through a process of indigenisation. They see opportunities to shape Western social work to fit with local values and norms (Atal, 1981; Bar-On, 2003; Cheung & Liu, 2004; Yunong & Xiong, 2008; Mandal, 1989; Tsang & Yan, 2001; Weaver, 1998, 1999, 2008; Yan & Tsui, 2007). Gray and Hetherington (2013) took indigenisation to mean that

> social work knowledge should arise from within the culture, reflect local behaviours and practice, be interpreted within a local frame of reference, and thus be locally relevant, that is it should address culturally relevant and context specific problems.
>
> (p. 27)

Khinduka (1971) believed indigenisation gave rise to confrontation, advocacy, coalition building, and political action for socioeconomic reform in the Global South. Ling

(2008) from Malaysia believed it involved an understanding of extended family networks, culture, religion, and spirituality and the theory of human development. She believed ethnographic and grounded approaches were most suitable for the development of locally relevant knowledge. Several Indian social workers connect indigenisation to *Sarvodaya*, a popular Indian movement initiated by Gandhi against the British aimed at economic and social reform (Kulkarni, 1993; Mandal, 1989; Nagpaul, 1993; Nanavathy, 1993; Nimmagadda & Chakradhar, 2006; Nimmagadda & Cowger, 1999; Rao, 2012). Cuban social workers are 'agents of community transformation', who engage in mobilising communities to analyse and address their own needs and problems (de Urrutia Barroso & Strug, 2013).

Local and cultural responses: Adaptive Global South

This approach seeks to adapt Western social work practice to local needs (Payne, 1997). Adaptation involves three stages: (i) Transmission – transfer of Western social work, (ii) indigenisation – attempts to adapt Western social work, (iii) and authentisation – an attempt to make it genuine within local contexts (Ragab, 1995, 2017; Walton & Nasr, 1988). As such, adaptation was a process of shaping social work to adapt to local political and sociocultural contexts (Walton & Nasr, 1988). It involves re-engineering micro and macro social work models, skills, and techniques to fit local structures and practice experience (Mukundarao, 1969). Ragab (1982, 1990, 2017) observed that, for Arab countries in the Middle East, indigenisation involved acknowledging a society's authentic roots in religion, language, and tradition. To become authentic or genuine, social work had to be grounded in local values, cultures, needs, and problems (Walton & Nasr, 1988). Indigenisation was thus a bottom-up approach. Many scholars see indigenisation as adaption, making Western social work to fit non-Western contexts, which leads to locally relevant, culturally appropriate social work (Cheung & Liu, 2004; Ling, 2003, 2004, 2008; Nimmagadda & Balgopal, 2000; Osei-Hwedie, 2002; Ragab, 1995; Shawky, 1972; Walton & Nasr, 1988; Wong, 2002; Yan & Cheung, 2006; Yan & Tsui, 2007; Yip, 2005a). The solution is seen 'authentisation' or 'contextualisation' of social work (Gray et al., 2008a; Hodge & Nadir, 2008; Hurdle, 2002; Midgley, 1981; Nanavathy, 1993; Osei-Hwedie, 2002; Ragab, 1982; Walton & Nasr, 1988).

Indigenous social work

Understanding the history of Indigenous Peoples, their closeness to the land, environment, and spirituality were prominent aspects of indigenous social work. Indigenous social work concerns Indigenous Peoples' rights and quest for justice (Gray et al., 2008b). Its political aims are:

> The development of healthy indigenous identities, increased participation in education, increased sociopolitical awareness, acquisition of research skills, preservation and reconnection to indigenous ways of knowing, opposition to stereotypes, identification of the community justice issues, engagement in social change efforts, changes in policy and structural oppressions, and contributions to public discourse on indigenous issue at the community, national, and international levels.
>
> (Johnston-Goodstar, 2013, p. 318)

Marais and Marais (2007) highlighted several aspects of indigenous world views. First, Indigenous People favour collective values – community, relationships, and connectedness – not only with other humans, but with all living and non-living species in their surrounding environment. Their holistic values are sharing, caring, and giving – respect for self, family, community, and nature, that is, benefitting the whole. Second, indigenous societies are polytheistic. Polytheistic religions include Hinduism, Mahayana Buddhism, Confucianism, Taoism, Shintoism, tribal religions in the Americas and Africa, and modern religious movement – neopaganism. With the exception of Christianity, Judaism, and Islam, most world religions are characterised by polytheism. Likewise, Mafile'o (2008) in New Zealand noted Tongan society valued experiences and relationships. Therein, Indigenous or culturally sensitive social work involved *Pola* (communal activity), *Fetokoni'aki* (mutual helping), *Faka'apa'apa* (respect), and *Ofa* (love).

Indigenous social work in the Global South

Indigenous social work in the Global South must be seen against the backdrop of colonisation and externally driven development, and their tendency to overlook traditional cultures. In Asian, Arab, and African societies, ethnicity, and religion are closely intertwined.

Hinduism's central tenets *dharma, karma,* and *moksha* heavily influence Nepali and Indian societies and inspire their members for the duty to one another, which, in other words, is a humanistic value. *Karma* is the fatalistic notion that a person's past actions and present life determines his or her future; what you give out you get back. Thus, poverty and suffering are the result of *karma* (Nimmagadda & Cowger, 1999). A good *dharma* and *karma* lead a person towards *moksha* (salvation). In Buddhism, the meaning of life and suffering are central; suffering is the route to enlightenment.

In Confucianism, a collective, relational orientation is given priority. It leads people to value their families more than their own personal goals, interests, and welfare (Yang, 1995). In Chinese culture, natural elements, such as *fung shui* (water and wind), *yin* and *yang* (shadow and sun), and *wui hang* (metal, wood, water, fire, and earth) control people's lives (Yip, 2002).

Despite modernisation and globalisation, these religious ideologies influence peoples' day-to-day lives. Most societies in the Global South value collectivism over individualism (Yip, 2005b). Nepal was a Hindu state until the peoples' movement overthrew the last monarch, King Gyanendra in 2007. Though now a secular nation, Hinduism and Buddhism still have a major influence on most peoples' lives.

In Arab societies, the Quran provides the basis for Muslim communities rooted in mutually interdependent relationships (Barise, 2005) and some Arab societies value human rights (Al-Dabbagh, 1993; Al-Krenawi & Graham, 1996, 2001; Barise, 2005; Haj-Yahia, 1997). However, there is uneasy fit between social work values and Islamic religious ideology, especially regarding women's rights (Holtzhausen, 2011; Ragab, 2017).

Judaism is part of social work's religious heritage, with social work rooted in Judeo-Christian values of respect, freedom, autonomy, independence, and social justice (Al-Krenawi & Graham, 2008). Zoabi and Savaya (2012) believe social work in Israel needs to reframe issues in culturally familiar terms and strategies, which would be easier to implement in practice.

Yip (2005a) distinguishes several characteristics of Chinese communities. First, Chinese communities are highly diversified. Most remote communities are traditional and free from modern influences. Second, Chinese culture does not have homogenous standpoints. Classical religious ideologies (Confucianism, Taoism, and Buddhism) and modern political ideologies (of Maoism, Marxism, and Leninism) have had strong impacts in China. Western ideologies, such as capitalism, materialism, and democracy are rapidly transforming Chinese society, however.

A paradigm shift from indigenisation to decolonisation

Decolonisation arises from the encounter between the history of Indigenous Peoples and the civilising mission of colonisation. It is a history of struggle and oppression, of ethnocide and political control. Decolonisation would like to tell Indigenous Peoples' stories, write their own version of history, and their struggle against colonialism or hegemonic Western approaches. As shown in Figure 5.2, decolonisation worldview in social work applies many of the concepts that emerged in relation to indigenous social work, discussed above.

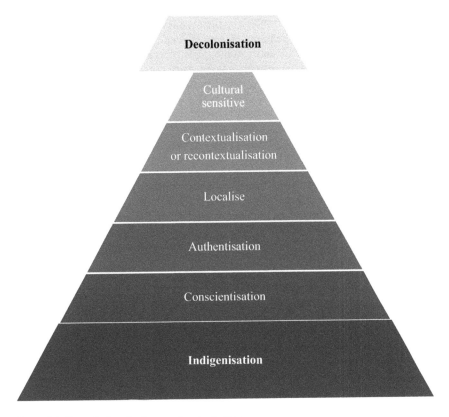

Figure 5.2 From indigenisation to decolonisation

As Wilmer (1993) proposed, Indigenous Peoples 'represent the unfinished business of decolonization' (p. 5). Broadly speaking, decolonisation involves deconstructing the effects of colonialism and imperialism. It is the act of reordering, recollecting, reclaiming, and reconstituting the lives of indigenous and colonised peoples (Smith, 2012). It means giving voice to marginalised groups and Indigenous People, silenced by colonialism. Yellow Bird (2008, 2013) explains,

- Many nation states have colonised indigenous lands; they have not only claimed territory, but also robbed Indigenous Peoples' of their cultural and social rights, and sovereignty.
- Colonial policies, and settler governments and agencies, have subjugated Indigenous Peoples through genocide, ethnocide, ecocide, and linguicide.

Despite scholarship on decolonisation in the social sciences, social work has been slow in developing its own theory. Gray et al. (2013c) conceptualised decolonisation in social work in terms of theory (thinking about indigenous social work), practice (from the bottom-up), education (facilitating local relevance), and research (decolonising methodologies). For Osei-Hwedie (1993), decolonisation involves the reclamation of cultures. Awareness of the decolonisation discourse enables social workers to withdraw from colonising projects (Gray et al., 2013c). Decolonisation is concerned with not only indigenous populations, but also non-Indigenous Peoples affected by global problems, such as climate change, pollution, poverty, and hunger that result from modernising development in the Global South (Wilson, 2013). Its goal is to 'protect and restore Indigenous Peoples' territories, natural resources, sacred sites, languages, beliefs, values, relationships, system of governance, sovereignty, self-determination, human rights and intellectual property' (Gray et al., 2013b, p. 5). As Smith (2012) observed, 'Decolonization, however, does not mean and has not meant a total rejection of all the theory or research or Western knowledge' (p. 41).

At heart, decolonisation is a political project. It asks, 'How can social work . . . contribute to social change when most social workers choose not to recognize the political dimensions of their practice and when political activism is not expressly advocated through social work professional bodies?' (Briskman, 2008, p. 83). Decolonisation is antithetical to modernist, consumerist, and materialistic ways of life (Rao, 2013). It calls for social workers to discard theoretical and practical frameworks that are harmful to Indigenous Peoples (Briskman, 2008).

Conclusion

The relationship between indigenisation and decolonisation delineated how decolonisation worldview has extended calls for cultural and local relevance to the political project; not only of reclaiming culture, but also of land rights and sovereignty for marginalised groups and Indigenous Peoples. Having reviewed the literature and set the context for the paradigm shift, Chapter 6 explores a ground-up experiences of Nepali social workers beginning with their motivation to choose social work education as well as their concerns surrounding around social work education and practice fit to Nepali society and its diverse social issues.

Influence and context for decolonised and developmental Nepali social work

Using bottom-up approach grounded in local cultures and contexts, this chapter rigorously builds the case for the decolonised and developmental Nepali social work. *Inter alia*, it empirically presents the competing dichotomy between the profession's Western hegemony on Nepali social work and the emerging local discourses rooted in Nepali socioeconomic, cultural, and political contexts. The chapter begins with participants' motivations. Then, it presents participants views on social work education and practice; the unique features of Nepali society that distinguish it from Western society; the social issues to which Nepali social workers are attempting to respond; the development-related activities in which they are engaged; and the issue of marginalisation and the need for political bent social work education and practice in Nepal.

Social workers' motivations

Participants believed social workers had a moral responsibility to contribute to Nepali society and to help others. Their humanistic worldview and interest in helping others had drawn them to social work. Some, like Kiran, had been involved in organising social activities, such as clean-up and blood donation campaigns prior to studying social work. He was motivated by the good he could do for others: 'When I see people's life being changed because of my contribution, it motivates me to do the things that I am doing now'. Volunteering had also inspired Niti and Sujit to become social workers. Sujit's observations had led him to believe,

> Many people are driven by passion. Regardless of their background, they think they must contribute to the betterment of the society. This [passion] guides us. Social bond is universal here. To help to the fellow citizen and contribute in the society is in our gene.

For him and others, like Niharika, Samikshya, and Urmila, their family and social surroundings motivated them to study social work. As Niharika explained,

> My family has always taught me to give back to the society. Therefore, I wanted to study something related to society. . . . I wanted to work for women and children. I have seen many women getting marriage at early age. Some of them are younger to me. I wanted to contribute in some ways. Therefore, I became social worker.

Urmila said,

> I joined social work education thinking I will be able to contribute to the society and make people independent. Since I am from outside of Kathmandu valley, where things are different, I have seen some of the severe problems in our locality. For instance, dowry system, [though legally not allowed, it continues as a social practice]. Mostly women are victims of such practice. I believed being a social worker I can bring changes in such system and contribute to women's lives.

Unlike others, for Niti and Samikshya, it was their practice experiences that had motivated them to continue social work practice:

> What I am today is not only the result of [my] educational background but also because of continued interactions with target groups, colleagues, stakeholders, as well as obtaining training from organisations. These all have shaped what I am today.
> (Niti)

Samikshya said she had been motivated by her practice experience rather than her social work education:

> If I evaluate my work, then I am happy. But if you are asking me in relation to my qualification, I do not find my educational background has any connection to the work that I am doing today. . . . In fact, some of educational teaching confront my work. For example, we were told in class not to be attached with target groups and always establish formal relationship with community. This way, it is difficult to work with Nepali communities where relationship is very informal.

Concerns about Nepali social work education

Motivation to contribute to Nepali society notwithstanding, the participants expressed concerns about the relevance of their social work education to the work they were doing. Kiran believed that social work education had been contaminated by Western ideas that had colonised the minds of Nepali social workers:

> Today's social work is very much attracted to Western philosophy. It's being glamourised. We were supposed to reflect our past, learn from there and make Nepali social work theory, but this is not happening. . . . On top of that, we as social workers of this country advocate [for] Western knowledge.

Similarly, Ranjan said, 'Many of the tools, methods, and practice guidelines are not suitable to the current context of the country. Maybe, with the expansion of modernisation and Westernisation, those might make sense here later'. Samikshya believed it was unlikely that Nepali people would seek the services of a social worker as this was foreign to their culture:

> That looked great while we were in social work class. Nobody will sign contract paper to engage self with social worker. Yes, we do sign some documents with our target group . . . while sanctioning loan to them through cooperatives. But, not

as defined in our education to make them client. . . . In my work, I do not apply even 'C' of casework. Most of work is different than casework. There are large groups of beneficiaries. We cannot afford casework. Again, our objective is different in the sense we are looking for mass empowerment and awareness. I wrote so many reports about casework while I was student, but they have no relation with my existing roles.

Urmila believed some Nepali social workers were positive about their Western social work education as this enabled them to migrate overseas; Nepal was supplying human resources without any investment from prospective overseas employers:

We were mostly taught about British, American, and Indian social work history. I cannot exactly explain history of social work in Nepal. However, I think social work was borrowed from Western context. Social work has Western influence, which is why most of the social work graduates migrate overseas after completing their degree here. It seems like we are investing on Nepali social work graduates so that they can serve others. . . . This is bitter reality of social work in Nepal.

Furthermore, most participants saw social work education as *bideshi siksha*, that is, foreign-influenced and expressed ambivalence about walking the tight-rope between the need for insider-initiated social work, while still building onto, and maintaining, imported Western world views, theories, and practice models. There was some concern about the Western roots of, and influences on, social work education imported from foreign universities and its inability to respond to local developmental and organisational dynamics, and Nepal's sociopolitical context. Sujit noted the 'mushrooming social work institutions' across the country, which Kiran observed were offering 'social work education [that was] Western rooted'. Kiran continued, 'I do not think there is any social work theory that I am using in the practice . . . [because] . . . they are from Western contexts, which are definitely not relevant to Nepali context'. He clarified this further:

Like two parallel lines, social work education and social conditions are diverging from each other [rather] than converging at [a] common point. . . . Our education and social problems are facing opposite to each other [and] our society is completely different than what we were taught. There is nothing called step-by-step procedures to solve problems like we were taught in [the] problem-solving process.
(Kiran)

Niti, a former academic now in practice, highlighted how Western psychologised social work was easy to teach but difficult to practice in Nepali communities:

Earlier I worked in academia. It was easy for me to teach social work in classroom setting. However, once I started my career in practice setting, it was difficult to utilise the same theoretical knowledge that I studied and . . . taught in the past. To extent, concepts like social work principles, target system, [and] action system can be related in the field. But, for example, we studied psychology and blah blah are never applied in the field . . . we studied about psychodynamic theory. Where do we use this psychological theory in our community work? We analyse people behaviour from our own perspective [culturally and socially informed] rather psy-chologically informed.

(Niti)

Indeed, she expressed sadness about Nepali social work education's inability to embrace a 'local reform approach':

> Our teacher taught us about Gandhian non-violent movement but they never talked about my previous organisation which has been applying non-violent approach and leading the landless peoples' movement for last 20 years. They have developed unique contextual approach that we as social workers do not know. We have never studied about local activists who sacrificed their life for peasants' rights. But we studied about many outsiders.

(Niti)

Believing that social work knowledge ought to be practice oriented, Namita reflected on social work education's theoretical focus: 'Social work is all about interacting with people – a practice approach, which cannot be understood merely through theoreti-cal underpinnings'. Therefore, she doubted whether Western 'theoretically overloaded social work education' would work in Nepali society.

Referring to development and the INGO where he worked, Ritesh expressed simi-lar concerns: 'Bilateral, multilateral, and government's policies . . . are not present in . . . social work contents'. Niharika noted that her social work education had not prepared her for work in a development agency: 'Technical skills, such as . . . report writing, monitoring, and evaluation, problem formulation, [and] logical framework analysis are not the foci of social work teaching'. Ranjan continued,

> Social work education does not fully prepare one person to work in [a develop-ment] agency because it has not covered each aspect of [development] practice settings . . . in [development] practice setting there are procedural things, such as organisational procedures and protocols, which are not covered in social work education.

Urmila referred to the failure of social work education to address and convey knowl-edge about the sociopolitical aspects of Nepali society:

> Knowledge about culture, caste, class, social institutions, history, relevant laws and policies, [including] currently changing natures of Nepali society was lacking in the social work curriculum. Also, social work education has not extensively cov-ered . . . local issues . . . we had rare discussion about caste-and geography-based discriminations in our classroom.

As highlighted by some participants, the question of social work education's rel-evance also related to the English language being imposed on social work students. As Niharika noted, 'We had to write all reports and exams in English. Only class discussion sometimes used to be in Nepali. It was something like English was dominant language, or say official language of social work'. It was difficult to translate borrowed social work terminology into localised and contextualised languages for use in practice. As Samikshya explained,

While interacting with community people, I used to use English terminologies. It used to be problematic because most of the community people do not understand English. I used to say 'problem' instead of saying *samasya*. Beneficiaries could not understand and used to ask what does that mean. I have not overcome it. Until now, I mix half English and half Nepali in the field. Many social work terminologies do not have exact translation in Nepali. It's [a] pity, *haina ra?*

This was especially difficult for the many students who had not gone to private boarding schools, where they would have learnt English at an early age. Above all, language barriers obstructed their ability to express themselves in the social surroundings in which they interacted. As Urmila explained,

> English and Nepali were communicative language [in BSW]. We had to produce fieldwork reports in English. Even exams were conducted in English. Coming from rural background and having studied in public school, I faced a lot of problems to express myself in English. Sometimes I could not express my opinion clearly in English.

Thus, for Samikshya, becoming a social worker was a sort of double burden as she had to relearn everything in the field:

> If we [can] integrate our social, cultural, and historical dynamics into social work, we will have maximum benefit. It will reduce burden of social work graduates from double learning process. Now we learn one thing in education and in the practice, we will have to again learn some other things. It will be easier for social workers to work in the field if we teach about actual social conditions in classrooms. The practice context will not look strange or new to social work graduates.

For Urmila, this was because 'the syllabus of Nepali social work education, [was] . . . merely replication of Western universities' that eschewed 'details about grassroots conditions' (Niharika). For Niharika, Nepali social work drew heavily on Western literature that had no connection to the Nepali social world:

> [The literature is] from outside, mostly from the USA and the UK. Few are from Indian context. Our library is full of foreign literatures. There are no books available relevant to Nepali context. This has also contributed in social work's slow progress in Nepal because we have been not able to generate our own literature.

When asked whether she had referred to Nepali literature, Samikshya replied adamantly, 'No! No! No! all the literatures came from outside. Theories, principles of social work, let say everything was developed by outsiders and we are so much accustomed to them'. She continued,

> I am not able to relate . . . [borrowed] educational training at all. My role relates to social and economic empowerment of women in rural areas. My organisation focuses on rural women's rights, especially improvement in economic lives of rural women. Nepal is still patriarchal society. [In most cases,] men control economic means. We believe [in our organisation that] even women can lead better

economic provided by equal opportunity and access to the resources. To work in such structural society, more than educational training, I have been applying life experiences to work with target groups. I think education was one thing and my work is another thing.

(Samikshya)

Sujit likewise questioned whether theories 'initiated outside' should 'influence our work or the work [initiated inside] should influence [our] theories'. Believing the latter, he concluded, 'We have enough culturally rooted knowledge – initiated inside – that has yet to be explored and, thus be used to craft future social work education in Nepal'. For Sujit, the interview had offered 'very important insights' and raised the question of what social work education ought to be.

The term knowledge economics aptly encapsulated the participants' perspectives on foreign-influenced social work education in Nepal. It refers to the neoliberal project that critical theorists maintain furthered the interests of the wealthy classes. It is a paradigm that seems to fit the participants' experiences in Nepal, given poor rural populations do not have access to higher education. For example, Kiran claimed,

> Private institutions are running [social work] course to which rural poor population do not have access. Plainly, they cannot afford as the tuition fee is relatively higher than other discipline. . . . For private educational institutions, social work education is a business.

Reflecting on access to education, Sujit, too, saw the dominant elitist ideology of private social work education as out of the reach of many marginalised Nepali populations, especially the rural poor. The system had systematically excluded them from entry into social work education and practice, by positioning the profession within the grip of a few urban elites, as Sujit explained, 'Only rich people, upper class and upper-middle class, . . . with lots of money or land, . . . can access social work education. [Also], mainly people of Kathmandu have access to [social work] education'.

Kiran believed most students came 'from urban centres of the country' and noted these urban-elite social work graduates were highly ambitious and career oriented and either remained in the capital city, Kathmandu, or moved overseas. Urmila, too, noted, 'Many graduates have already migrated overseas. They studied so that they can migrate abroad for better lives'; and Ritesh observed,

> Although rural areas must be target for social workers, we do not want to be placed there because there is neither opportunity nor facility. You want to build your career. If social workers stay in Kathmandu, they have more access to the resources.

Sujit believed, 'Rural people should be given the opportunity to study social work so that they will apply social work interventions to deal with their challenges back to their original places'. For this to eventuate,

> either government or social work institutions must create scholarship [programs] for rural population to study social work. . . . Educational institutions . . . [ought to] focus on holistic quality of social work education [rather] than simply increasing the numbers of graduate merely for economic benefit.

Participants also questioned social work educators' pedagogical methods and lack of familiarity with, and exposure to, local practice settings. Some educators trained in Western countries could not relate their 'outside knowledge' to the Nepali context and used professional jargons that were incomprehensible to many Nepali social work students. Kiran remembered his educator thus:

> Our teacher . . . was trained in the USA. She used to give example of social workers counselling parents accused of corporal punishments. In Nepali society, it is common and justified. She could have given Nepali-related examples. . . . Those who teach us, even they lack [critical, spatial] knowledge. They are trained in international universities, use big terminologies, glittery words, and jargons . . . which are not applicable to Nepali society.

Other educators teaching social work were not formally trained social workers. Reflecting on the quality of social work educators, Kiran observed, 'They are from other related disciplines, such as psychology, sociology, anthropology, and so forth. . . . I doubt what kind of quality of social work education they usher'. Niharika remarked, 'Even teachers are not clear what they are teaching'. Ritesh said, 'If you want me to be honest, those teachers are not qualified to teach us. They are not social work graduates. They share knowledge from their discipline'. Above all, these educators had yet to develop and embrace local pedagogical methods in teaching social work.

Participants believed that locally relevant social work education would be diversity oriented, since Nepal comprised diverse populations. Kiran suggested, 'It is imperative that social work education reflects . . . [Nepali peoples'] lives at one hand and address their contemporary social challenges on the other hand. [It should] intend to address regional diversity of the country'. Sujit believed, 'Multicultural, multilingual, and diversity sensitive education' was needed. Niharika added, it must include political debates within its contents as 'at the end . . . [social workers] affiliate with NGOs, CBOs and GOs [government organisations], which are very political in nature' and often, 'social workers have to engage in advocacy and activism' that require a sound comprehension of political discourses.

Samikshya believed there was no need to confine social work students within the boundary of borrowed Western social work principles and prospects. Rather, she advocated the inclusion of surrounding social realities in social work education:

> We write reports after every field visit. We have been told to relate with [Western] theoretical knowledge, which, according to me, is not a good practice. The moment, we confine ourselves we cannot think beyond those theoretical frameworks. It is not necessary that we use the terminologies that have been borrowed from somewhere else. Students should be encouraged to reflect what they have observed, what they have felt in relation to community . . . these things have to be adapted in course of contents.
>
> (Samikshya)

Participants saw a need to adapt social work knowledge to local 'beneficiary groups', as Samikshya outlined:

> When we are working with beneficiary groups, we come to know about many perspectives. If we can blend those experiences in our education, social work will

be effective. We come to know about problem, as well as solution, from beneficiary groups.

Ranjan believed that Nepali social work education should equip social work students with practical knowledge, not just broader theoretical perspectives:

> While designing curriculum, the authorities must reflect practice contexts. For example, there is one course called 'paralegal' [work]. Social workers require knowledge of practice-related laws, such as relating to children and women, [rather] than general laws. Social work students are supposed to be equipped with the concept of human rights violations and subsequent legal remedies . . . [many] social work students do not have knowledge where a child labour case should be reported. They are oblivious to Labour Office of Nepal.

A practice-oriented education would lead to better understanding of practice settings and subsequent problem-solving skills. Moreover, students would be confident to work in development agencies, as noted by Namita. Social work education should strengthen students' 'analytical skills' (Ritesh) and 'capacity' (Sujit) to work in any social conditions and contexts.

Concerns about professional elitism

Participants saw social work as *sukila mukila pesha*, that is, bourgeois or elitist and wondered whether it could truly solidify around poor people's concerns. As Sujit observed, 'The rich people study social work to help poor peoples of Nepal'. Urmila believed, 'By doing social work, I have changed my [socioeconomic] status but not [that] of the community for which I work'. Observing that most social workers were from privileged families – in terms of high class, caste, or situation in urban areas – Niharika claimed, 'The country's worsening scenarios do not disturb social workers'. Kiran believed that, for many, becoming a social worker meant safeguarding their membership in an elite club:

> Social work is run by rich people to educate rich people who want to work for poor people. Isn't this irony? . . . These rich social workers follow Western fashion and go to the fields [communities], where people feel uncomfortable to their dresses. Until now, rural populations consider Western fashions inappropriate. But, social workers of Nepal neglect this reality. Recently, rural people can identify social workers working in INGOs by the kind of dress they wear, which is expensive and on fashion trend. [For many] becoming a social worker and then working in an INGO in this country is a sort of gaining entry to elite-brand.

In addition, Kiran believed Nepali social work had yet to decide its *raison d'etre* in Nepali society:

> I want to use a term to . . . [describe social work in Nepal], that is, glamorisation. This is a big problem of Nepali social workers. High salary expectation [and] urban accessibility all social workers want here. Social workers want geographical feasibility as well. . . . [They] are not glamorised by themselves. It is NGOs and

INGOs, social work institutions, and our formal or informal affiliations to international universities are contributing to the glamorisation of social work. . . . In comparison to other disciplines, social work students are portrayed in glamorised and glittery way even inside colleges and universities.

A few participants indicated how social work was just becoming a talking profession rather than one working and contributing to Nepali society. For example, both Kiran and Samikshya mentioned social workers' excessive concern with gaining professional status in the country. In fact, Samikshya described imported social work as a profession that 'talks the talk but does not walk the walk'. Sujit saw Nepali social workers losing their long-established social norms of volunteerism and benevolence:

> Historically and traditionally social work has been considered as [a] vocation in Nepal . . . [but] when it comes to social work as [a] profession, passion may or may not drive social workers to contribute in the society. For example, as a social worker, I might work in an organisation for two years or, let's say five years. But given the good offer by any other organisation, I will move from here. I will be least bothered about the organisation, including the people with whom I have been working currently.

For Tulshi, the cloak of professionalism had led to a loss of vocation yet she was sceptical about those working with community groups, who were not formally trained, that is, who did not have a social work education. Many Nepali social workers saw professional growth in terms of upward mobility, mainly concerning to personal benefit – better salaries and positions:

> From the very beginning, we are told social work is a profession, we need to earn from it. Therefore, we . . . emphasise immediate [personal] benefit . . . in terms of cash or facilities [rather] than benefiting the community peoples. . . . It's [a kind of] individual or family investment. Naturally, they expect immediate return.
>
> (Sujit)

Ritesh believed that this professional extremism was harmful. Citing the example of an NGO solely founded and run by social workers, he criticised their narrow concept of development and conscious exclusion of related disciplines. Further, he argued, 'Whether we are professional social workers or development practitioners, we need to think broader. We must implement social work's worldview but, at the same time, we have to also consider others . . . [working in] GOs, NGOs, and INGOs' (Ritesh) to make the development field holistic and sustainable.

Niharika believed that social workers 'haven't served in Nepali society', while Kiran thought this was because 'we do not know many things about Nepali society. What is happening in the society? What is the structure of the society? These are unknown territory for us'. In other words, social work had yet to make Nepali people feel its presence, especially, when it came to serving rural and remote areas and vulnerable and marginalised populations in the country:

> [Social workers] are not able to reach to grassroots locations and address their basic needs. . . . Grassroots require social workers than any urban locations. . . . Frankly,

we do not want to change society. We do not want to visit rural areas because working in rural areas is difficult and challenging.

(Kiran)

Sujit explained how social work has neglected bottom section of the society:

There are many [development] organisations, programs, and activities addressing the issues of marginalisation in Nepal. However, they are not from professionally trained social work background. In other words, marginalised people are out of reach of social workers' services. . . . To reach out to the marginalised people is not the priority of Nepali social workers. . . . Until now social work institutions are centralised to Kathmandu. . . . [Hence] social workers have never reached to the people and place at the bottom of the society . . . [because its] education has not sufficiently encouraged social workers to work at grassroots level.

Ranjan referred to borrowed social work's insensitivity and unsuitability to Nepali society as it was 'designed to fit . . . Western nations [that] are resting on individualism and are already developed'. Urmila believed social workers had yet to work out 'what exactly [they] are going to do in the society'. Since social workers had yet to determine the kind of agencies they were going to work in; the nature of their activities and profession; and how they were going to position themselves in relation to their target groups, several participants expressed their frustration: 'I am neither too satisfied nor too disappointed [being a social worker] . . . to the extent what I wanted to contribute being a social worker is not happening' (Kiran) and 'being a social worker I do not know the real situations of country. I cannot confidently claim [that] I am a social worker because I lack knowledge to understand Nepali society and social problems' (Urmila).

From his experiences of working in an INGO and academia, Ranjan said there was no way to comprehend 'what kind of social worker is being produced . . . there is no quality control. Social work is just messed up . . . social work graduates should be worried . . . if they want to protect their profession'. Sujit added he was oblivious to 'what is happening in social work field [as] there is no proper study being conducted'. He continued pessimistically, 'We are going to end nowhere in the future'.

What the 'social' in Nepali 'social work' entails: the case for decolonisation

The unique features of Nepali society that emerged from the participants' perspectives were grouped into five dimensions of the 'social'. They included the:

1   Contra-distinction between Nepali society and the Western worldview.
2   Social cohesion, the ties that bind.
3   Social fabric, that is, Nepali social workers' understanding of everyday social phenomena that guide, control, and dominate Nepali peoples' interpersonal interactions.
4   Structural diversification refers to the complex structure and regional variation of Nepali society.
5   Dynamic normative refers to the historically and culturally established norms and institutions of Nepali society.

Contra-distinction between Western and Nepali society

Urmila believed Nepali society was 'completely different from Western society'. In the first instance, Nepali understanding of the 'individual' was quite unique, as Kiran explained. The notion of the 'individual' was a

> collective construct . . . shaped by the broader interactions of family, society, peer groups [and so on] . . . when we consider foreign country, we take individual as single unit but in Nepal an individual is not an individual . . . [but] totally a collective [product].
>
> (Urmila)

Urmila, who was born in a rural part of Nepal and completed her university studies in Kathmandu, well understood the notion of the 'collective individual'. Her experience travelling to different parts of Nepal as a social worker employed by an INGO led her to believe that Nepali people were 'always eager to help each other. If an individual is facing problem, then entire family and [sometimes even the] community come together to help her' (Urmila). Neither the problem nor its solutions remained solely the responsibility of the individual; as elsewhere, what an individual in Nepali society became was the product of family and social influences to instil a collective sense of personhood. Niharika put it, 'We are not like Western people. In their society "I" [and] "self" rule [rather] than "we"'. This extended to social practices, as Urmila explained:

> When we go to restaurant we do not bother about who will pay. We do not have 'getting together and paying self' kind of approach like many Western people have. We do not divide bill at restaurant. It is always a person steps forward to pay the bill. Also, we share foods at restaurant and do not just eat what we order individually. It is a bit uncomfortable every time I go to restaurant with expats.

Second, this concept of collective individuality had a bearing on the understanding of human rights in Nepali society. Rather than an expression of individual freedom, as they were understood in the Western world, in Nepal, rights were collective and socially negotiated. Kiran used the example of corporal punishment, which, despite of its illegal status remained socially acceptable in Nepal, but, in the USA, would be viewed as a violation of an individual's rights. Ranjan gave an example of divorce in Nepali society, which, until recently, was not common due to issues relating to child custody. If a couple should divorce, the family and community, not the parents who were divorcing, would decide custody issues. They rarely became a legal matter. From a rights perspective, Nepali society upheld the child's right to a family, which also prevented child neglected.

Social cohesion of Nepali society

Participants considered the social cohesion of Nepali society lays in 'collectiveness' (Namita), 'surviving', 'communal feelings', 'mutual interdependence' (Ranjan), 'helping each other' (Niti), 'unity' (Samikshya), and 'togetherness' (Niharika). These strengths were embedded through festivals and rituals, such as *Kshama Puja* (forgiveness rituals) and *Bhumi Puja* (worship to earth), and traditional cultural practices, such as *guthi*, which were gradually fading away, however (Sujit). For centuries, Nepali people had been fulfilling their needs (through *guthi*), releasing their fear and emotions (through rituals), and simultaneously collectively expressing joy (through festivals). They embedded the binding value of 'unity in diversity', as Niharika explained:

> We believe in communal feelings rather than individualisation. So, Nepali society means togetherness, mutual sentiments, [and] 'we-feeling'. . . . Unity in diversity defines Nepali society. There are many ethnic groups, many linguistic groups but there is togetherness [to an extent] among them.

These strengths promoted an ethic of care within families and neighbourhoods. As Kiran explained, 'In Nepal there is no [institutional] practice of personal caregiver even in the case of disability. People are cared [for] by their families, relatives, including sometimes by neighbours'. For Niti, 'the value of Nepali society rests upon helping each other', a value that had sustained human civilisations everywhere throughout history.

Social fabric

By social fabric is meant the participants' understanding of factors that shaped Nepali social interaction, such as understandings of time, cultural boundaries, and dominant 'we-feeling' world views. Niti described Nepali people's sense of time as 'let's do it gradually', reflecting their attitude of continuous reflection and lifelong learning. As Niti explained, from her experience,

> Our development pace is slower because of our belief [in gradual progress] . . . we do not have rapid development. . . . One of our partner community-based organisations has been working in the issue of landless for last 20 years. People are not hopeless. They continue to believe [that] one day they will achieve their goal, but their pace is very slow. They do not shift from one approach to another radically.

Influenced by her Western education, Niti thought, at times, people should be pressurised to accelerate the pace of development but was aware this might create dependency. Ranjan described Nepali people as patient in their belief that someday things would change for the better:

> People are resilient. People can cope with devastations either manmade (sic) or natural. Within a few days of earthquake [on April and May 2015], they have come back to normalcy. They are also patience even at a time when government is not able to fulfil its duties. There are unmanaged potholes on roads for long time. Government has taken no measures to fix them. If someone falls there, we do not take it as failure of government accountability. Rather, we stand up, clear dirt and go home.

Samikshya believed that 'cultural boundaries' prevented her from adopting a Western lifestyle:

> Personally, even I cannot accept every Western ideal. I am well educated, have master degree in social work, but cannot accept all Western lifestyle, for example living relationship. Maybe I will say I am an open-minded person, but I am tied up with cultural, personal, and family limitations. I am a social worker but I am still traditional, to some extent.

She also talked about the central role of family:

> It is not like Western society where, after certain age, an individual is free from parents or family. In Nepali society, family continues to have close bonds with individuals. Family sponsors individual's education and fulfil other needs, such as economic.
>
> (Samikshya)

In Nepal, the social world was built around service to others, ritual, and nature. As Niharika explained, '*dharma* and *karma*' constructed '*pati-pauwa* [and] *kuwa* for community welfare' in the past. The very concept of doing social work was already present in 'the social world' of Nepali people eliminating the need to borrow social work from elsewhere. Rituals and nature 'helped people to control emotions and fears' (Ranjan). Participants believed some exceptions within the social world had long threatened Nepali society, such as the 'tendency to follow outsiders without thinking' (Kiran) and 'copying others without realising whether that will be sustainable and productive [and] . . . doubting integrating past . . . [in] development thinking' (Sujit). This also meant the social fabric of Nepali society was fragile and likely to be eroded with global influences at any time.

Structural diversification

The structural diversification of Nepali's heterogeneous and complex social structures, such as caste and class (Kiran), regional variations, such as *Himali*, *Pahade*, and *Madheshi* (Ritesh), and rural and urban areas (Sujit), its pluralistic society (Urmila), and diverse cultures created a multilayered society. Participants referred to 'different lifestyles' (Niti) and 'cultural diversity' (Urmila), while Niti noted 'the differences amongst Western, far-Western, and Eastern regions' that had significant impacts on peoples' lives: 'People's lifestyles are different to each other. [Geography] . . . has great effect in their lifestyle. Likewise, even social issues are different there'. Structural diversification made for hierarchy, dominance, and oppression:

> In resource access caste, class, and gender play a significant role. Those who are in upper caste and upper class strata can easily influence state and non-state mechanism, and thus equip them with the available resources. Sometimes they would create resources for them.
>
> (Kiran)

This compromised social work's broad goal of promoting human worth and dignity for all. However, Niharika believed that social workers were oblivious to these injustices, since they were not discussed extensively in the curriculum.

Dynamic normative

The dynamic normative dimension referred to historically and culturally established norms and institutions that shaped social life of Nepali people. With the advent of democracy,

> things are changing. . . . Social change is a process that will keep on happening. Whether it is nation's encounter to modernisation process or its adoption of new approaches in the name of progress or development; new insights will replace the traditional ones.
>
> (Sujit)

Further, Sujit claimed that several practices of his ethnic group including 'rituals, and festivals . . . [are] changing. . . . These are not the priority of people in modern era because of people's changing priorities, such as ambition to become rich [and] attain modern facilities'. As he noted, 'People are opting for nuclear family over joint family'. Likewise, Sujit observed, 'Rural push and urban pull was high in the country. People are moving to urban areas from rural areas'. He also mentioned that an erosion of the caste-based division of work had already changed people's 'ways of earning . . . whatever they prefer, they choose as an employment' (Sujit). Samikshya believed that, while 'there is bit of Westernisation and modernisation influence in Nepali society . . . intercaste marriage is gradually being accepted'. Nonetheless, resistance persisted as people 'haven't forgotten their tradition . . . they are not fully following modern lifestyle' (Samikshya).

Social issues for Nepali social work: the case for development

The dominant social issues mentioned by participants included:

- Poverty (Ranjan, Niharika, and Samikshya).
- Discrimination and oppression over minorities (Niharika).
- Landlessness (Niti).
- Girl trafficking (Samikshya).
- Child-related exploitation, such as child labour abuse, and violence (Ranjan), child abuse, corporal punishment, street children, and domestic child labour (Niharika).
- Gender issues, such as gender-related violence (Niti).
- Care of elderly people (Niharika).

However, the overriding issue was poverty (Niharika and Sujit). There was some agreement that the interrelated issues of poverty, social injustice, regional disparities, and systematic oppression and discrimination against minorities were structural (sociocultural) and political issues:

> There is systematic discrimination and oppression over minority groups in the society . . . minorities in terms of caste, geography, and disadvantaged groups. . . . Even, there are some reservation system or say positive discrimination, many [minorities] people who are entitled to it are not able to access [advantages] because of corruption and political influences.
>
> (Niharika)

'Traditions, norms, and conservative beliefs . . . [have caused] abundant problems in the country' (Kiran), especially in stereotyping lower caste groups (Niti) and women (Kiran, Samikshya, Urmila, and Niharika). Niti recognised, 'Untouchability [or casteism] is product of Nepali cultural practice . . . [that] cannot be radically changed'. In these multiple, interconnected problems (Ranjan), poverty was 'massive' (Samikshya):

> It is complex. There are multiple problems and they are . . . interconnected. For instance, street children in urban area are the result of poverty in rural areas. Increasing squatters in urban areas are again the result of lack of unemployment and poverty in rural areas. The faces of problems are different but they have similar origins. Many women have been trafficked outside of nation. Many migrated

Nepali youths have been exploited in Gulf nations. These all have common roots unemployment, poverty, and political instability of the country.

(Ranjan)

To this, Sujit reflected,

We intend to graduate from the least developed country soon. But that does not seem possible according to the current situation of the country. Low economic condition is still a primary social problem of the country . . . poverty is a big problem of our nation.

Many 'have been forced to migrate to the countries of Middle East and Malaysia' (Niharika) due to the state of crucial poverty. Many are deprived of 'accessing school. . . . People are poor, families are poor, and communities are poor. Everyone does not have access to development [goals and programs]' (Niharika), but structural or political solutions do 'not seem possible in the current situation of the country' (Sujit). Poverty was seen to be exacerbated by:

- 'The quality' (Ritesh) and 'access[ibility]' (Niharika) of education.

Lacking access to education has significant impacts on people's thinking and perception. Since [significant portion of populations] . . . are not educated, there is less opportunity for them. Our organisation's research is showing that people are fed up with education. Many of students are dropped out from secondary school because they see many university graduates unemployed in their communities. They think it's better to migrate to Gulf nations to earn (Ritesh).

Some had access but, overall, the quality of and accessibility to education was questionable: 'Many girls are deprived from schooling' (Niharika).

- Technical discrepancies (Niti, Namita, and Ranjan), that is, the government's failure to implement policies and plan, hence people lacked awareness of existing policies: 'Communities are not empowered to know, utilise, and engage policies of government' (Namita). 'In absence of technical arrangements, people have been taking care of themselves . . . there is no systematic government plan and policy to improve individual or public lives', Ranjan noted.
- Absence of policies on landlessness (Niti).

In terms of landless, government land policy is not effective. On top of that, government lacks serious efforts to . . . uplift landless people of the country. One government provides them temporary settlement, the next one chases them. This is like a cyclical process. Government has not given any solid and permanent solution to the issue of landless in the country (Niti).

- Discrimination against women.

Participants saw gender issues as the product of some of the Nepali sociocultural practices in which the dominant patriarchy was justified over gender equality and equity (Ranjan and Ritesh) and women lacked ownership of economic means (Niharika and Samikshya). Women were often accused of 'practising witchcraft' (Samikshya) and considered a burden because of the 'practice of dowry' (Niharika). For Niharika, 'traditional harmful practices, such as early girl marriage, *Chhaupadi Pratha*, [and] . . . discrimination on the basis of gender at home' resulted in males being given more preference to education and girls dropping out of school early, especially due to early marriage. Also, issues relating to sexual reproductive rights led to women giving birth to many children at an early age. From her experience of working with Nepali cross-cultural communities, Urmila illustrated the way in which culture had restricted women's roles and status by subordinating them in the family and in the society:

> There is lack of awareness [of sociocultural and political dynamics] amongst women. Moreover, there is traditional belief that women must stay at home. First, these women are under control of parents and then under the control of husbands. [Second,] women are not free here, which refrain them to grow in everyday life. We need to alter the belief that women are not capable. Our society compares women with ornaments, and [explicitly] advocates women should not step outside of home. This has to be changed (Urmila).

- The 'ideology of governance' (Ranjan).

This had contributed to the development of 'structural social issues' (Samikshya), such as Nepal's 'low economic profile, unemployment, [and] . . . uncontrolled market inflation' (Niharika). 'To intervene in people's problem, we should be aware of the governance system. What are the government ideologies'? According to Ranjan 'liberalisation and privatisation inform the government policies'. Further, he believed that Nepal's entry into globalisation and free trade threatened Nepali citizens' ability to escape dire poverty:

> People seek to address their poverty using their entrepreneurial skills, but sadly they cannot compete with the mass production. . . . To intervene peoples' problem, we should be also mindful to the governance system. What are the ideologies of government . . . liberalisation and privatisation. Also, we are already part of globalisation and free trade. It is hard to challenge the big business, which have mass productions. Empowering our target groups through entrepreneurial approach is not adequate to compete with big industries. Social workers have to consider this aspect while working to change peoples' lives.
>
> (Ranjan)

- Political instability.

This had hindered the country's ability to generate a progressive vision of economic and industrial development, which is essential for retaining its labour force and creating employment opportunities for the nation:

> There is political factor as well. Few years ago, Nepal had productive industries. Nepal Airlines and Thai Airways started [almost] same time. But you cannot compare these two now. Thai Airways is established than ours. Earlier our national industries had created adequate employments. What happened to them? All of them have collapsed. We are rich in hydropower. With the increasing populations, we were supposed to increase hydropower capacity that we did not do. Thus, we

have hours of blackout every day. Thus, in every possible way, [blame goes to Nepal's prolonged political instability that] . . . obstructed the means of productions, which resulted in unemployment. The mass migrant workers are the result of this only.

(Ranjan)

- Absence of a rights culture (Niharika).

There were certain Western practices some participants wanted to emulate, such as a rights culture but, for Niharika, the country had yet to manage and strengthen its democratic norms for sharing power and resources. People did not have voice and were not 'politically active and influencing' (Ranjan) in developments in mainstream society. Given myriads of macrolevel social issues in Nepal, participants believed framing social work intervention within development discourse was inevitable, which I explore in the following section.

Development as key mantra in Nepali social work

Bideshi sanstha (foreign institution) and bideshi vikash (foreign development)

In Nepali, *bideshi* means 'foreign', *sanstha* means 'institution', and *vikash* means 'development'. Hence *bideshi sanstha's vikash* refers to institutional development largely driven by foreign or international organisations. From the participants' perspectives, INGOs as *bideshi sanstha* played an increasing role in Nepali development.

Samikshya believed that INGO programs were more effective than the 'government's [own] efforts, that is, *swadeshi aadhar*' (discussed below). Niharika claimed her organisation benefitted families and communities by enhancing access to education, health, nutrition, and water provision. Poverty reduction was a major focus, though most of the organisations had multiple programs, including children's and women's rights advocacy, agricultural development and environmental sustainability, humanitarian relief, peace, and conflict management, self-help and livelihood support, and income generation:

> We have ranges of programs focused to issues such as disaster management, . . . socioeconomic empowerment of marginalised groups and rural population, interior place management related to agriculture, climate change, gender empowerment, conflict and peace management. . . . In general, we are community-based organisation.
>
> (Samikshya)

The main goal of *bideshi sanstha* was human development, in keeping with contemporary international development policy. Common terms included environmental sustainability, social capital, fair and just access to resources, fair treatment irrespective of gender and age, improved agriculture, good governance, and cooperation. Strategies being used included participatory and integrated approaches, community security model, volunteerism, and multidimensional poverty reduction through local partnership development (see Table 6.1). However, participants were also critical of these

Table 6.1 Development-related activities

Programs	Participant	Strategy
Access to 'education', 'health', 'nutrition', and 'water'	Niharika	• 'Participatory, integrated approach' (Samikshya)
Advocacy of children's and women's rights (to 'gender equality')	Niti, Samikshya, Niharika, Ranjan, Kiran	• 'Community security model' (Ritesh)
Agriculture 'interior place management for agriculture'	Samikshya	• 'Volunteerism', 'multidimensional poverty reduction
Empowerment and capacity building, especially 'social and economic empowerment'	Samikshya, Sujit	strategy', and 'need-based approach' (Sujit)
Governance, including policy implementation	Niharika	• 'Local partnership' (Niti)
Humanitarian 'disaster management and relief distribution'	Samikshya, Niharika	
Management of 'conflict and peace'	Samikshya, Ritesh	
Promotion of 'environment and climate'	Niti, Samikshya	
Self-help 'cooperatives'	Samikshya	
Support 'livelihoods', 'income generation', and 'poverty reduction'	Niharika, Sujit, Samikshya	

'self-praising organisations', their 'short-term impacts on communities', and their generation of a 'dependency mentality' among the Nepali population:

> *Bideshi sanstha* has made societies donor dependent. Until project is running in a particular area, you can see peoples' lives are changing. Once the project is over, people go back to the previous stage.
>
> (Niti)

> [*Bideshi sansthas*] . . . see their comfort. For instance, my organisation used to have programs in Doti and Achham, remote parts of the country, but we withdrew from there because of difficulty. We see our easiness. So, now we only run program to the places where there is transportation accessibility and we do not have to walk for long hours. . . . We are mostly involved in self-praising rather actually changing Nepali communities. . . . I feel sad when I find we are wasting our efforts, resources, and funding at wrong location.
>
> (Samikshya)

Sujit wondered, 'Who is driving social changes in the country? Is this internally initiated or some interest-group driven? Or, is there outsider's influence?' To him, the answer was clear: 'Development initiatives are funded, developed, and designed by outsiders . . . the notion of Nepali development inherent in and propagated by Western discourses' (Sujit). Samikshya, too, was 'not in favour that Nepal should rely on *bideshi vikash* – development from outside model' – that was trapping Nepali people into a vicious cycle of aid-dependency. Worrying to Ritesh was INGOs' influence on local agencies' plans and programs: 'Beneath their aid supplies, there are . . . vested interests, policies, and politics. Often, they also have preferential supply of aid. Local agencies receive aid from their links'. Niharika noted that *bideshi vikash* created employment opportunities for expats, who 'influence the programs [of local agencies] as the funds come from them, [while] in program implementation frontline workers are Nepali'. *Bideshi vikash* thus supported the political economy of colonisation and systematically excluded local stakeholders, who promoted popular development principles, such as participation, decentralisation, and self-reliance.

Participants agreed that a social worker must have basic technical understanding of development aid-related protocols and humanitarian activities, and program and organisational management. As Ranjan observed, social workers required technical knowledge related to organisations:

> In practice setting there are procedural things such as organisational procedures and protocols, which are not covered in social work education. . . . Organisation also requires employee to be sound about relevant policies and laws. Apart from basic knowledge of social work, we also require some technical knowledge to work in organisation.

INGO work required knowledge of 'approaches to development and poverty reduction'; 'national policies and laws' (Ranjan); and 'contextual knowledge about target [or beneficiary] groups' (Niti). Also, needed were skills in 'social and political analysis' (Namita), 'mobilising communities' (Niti), and 'planning, reporting, communicating, fundraising, and administration' (Niharika). Such knowledge and skills preparation were lacking in social work, where curricula were dominated by psychodynamic approaches to social work practice. As Tulshi noted, there was a 'mismatch between social work education and required skills in [development] organisations'. This undermined social workers' contribution within INGOs, as Samikshya and Ranjan observed:

> I am employed at the position of junior program coordinator under which reporting, field visits, technical supports to field staffs, contacting donors, develop proposals, and making strategic changes in program interventions are my current roles . . . but our syllabus is not compatible to . . . [those]. Plenty of things are psychology related, which will of course help if I want to work as counsellor, otherwise they are not relevant to organisation, which is developmental in nature.
> (Samikshya)

> Once I had to develop curriculum about early childhood development. I thought it would be easy as we were taught about developmental psychology. We knew about . . . early childhood development but we missed to explore what activities will ensure such development of child. What short of preschool programs should be there for children to enhance early childhood development? This was challenging for me.
> (Ranjan)

Due to their lack of development knowledge, 'INGOs do not give priority to social work graduates' (Niharika) and 'assume any social science graduates can serve their organisational goals' (Niti). In a rather lengthy explanation, Niharika observed,

> The organisation where I am working, which is established in more than 120 nations, and even working in Nepal for more than four decades, and also work in close collaboration with the government, has no more than four social work graduates as employees. My organisation has several issues, such as child protection, child rights, governance, humanitarian, livelihood, HIV, and other areas. But it has not employed social workers to contribute in those areas. If my organisation being donor does not recognise social worker, you can imagine the condition of social workers in the partner organisations, [that is, local CBOs and NGOs]. . . . It might happen because social work graduates do not have clear vision. They do not know how this discipline fit to Nepali development scenario. . . . If any social worker is already employed and has demonstrated competent skills in the organisation, they might recruit other social workers from the same educational institute but not because they are social workers. . . . They can be any social science graduates. . . . In other international branches of our organisations there are post for social workers, not in Nepal. May be my organisation does not think social work of Nepal are prepared to tackle . . . [developmental] issues.
>
> (Niharika)

The term *vikashi kura* literally means 'development debate'. Here it refers to the debate between top-down (foreign development) and bottom–up grassroots development 'within the communities' capacities' (Sujit). Grassroots development involved community-led, sustainable processes, responding to local needs, as Urmila explained:

> Communities, . . . local agencies . . . with government local bodies . . . organise community meetings to discuss about problems or issues [and] . . . ensure participation of gender, age, ethnicity, and other diversities . . . provide community people training so that they can address their problems by themselves.

Strategies included 'community development' (Samikshya), 'community organisation' (Sujit) – 'asset-based development' (Sujit), a 'need based approach' (Ritesh), and focused on social integration and social capital (Ranjan, Niharika, and Niti). *Bideshi sanstha* and *bideshi vikash* were seen to impede community-driven development, where local people took ownership of development, as Niti explained:

> There are some of the ownership-based groups, which have long-term development impacts. To the extent, they are sustainable. They believe that they do not require any external supports. They generate internal resources and try to influence local and central stakeholders through activism.

Swadeshi aadhar: Government in development

Here, *Swadeshi aadhar* used in terms of 'domestic or national government intervention' was perceived as a hurdle for development. The term was used to refer to the government's failure in development. Participants criticised the weak design of development policies and structures; problems in policy formulation and implementation; the lack of bureaucratic accountability; preferential treatment of citizens; inefficient and ineffective public sector management; and the government's inability to generate a strong economic base to support development expenditure. Samikshya was sceptical about putting government and development together and doubted that the government could respond effectively to development issues due to 'financial and technical constraints'. Kiran, too, criticised government development endeavours because of poor policies, nepotism, and favouritism that were embedded in the system and led to the poor becoming poorer:

> Caste, class, and gender play a significant role to access government resources. Those who are in upper caste and upper class strata can easily influence state and also easily connect themselves with the available resources . . . poor policy [is] forcing. . . poor to become poorer in the society . . . our government is not self-sufficient. . . . In addition, the social policies are elite informed that do not address many living at the grassroots.
>
> (Kiran)

Also, participants observed the government's failure to implement development initiatives due to institutional corruption in its top-to-bottom structures, as Urmila explained:

> [For policy implementation,] we have channels from ministry to . . . [local] level. But these have not been effectively implemented . . . government lacks monitoring and evaluation of its programs. For example, government provides certain budgets to each . . . [local level] annually. But how it is spent there is no proper monitoring and evaluation.

Likewise, Namita observed that the 'government is not concerned to execute its policies properly. There are no proper supervisions and monitoring of government's policies'. Consequently, it created a smokescreen under which corruption could easily breed. Thus, part of the constraints in development related to 'corrupt ministers and politicians' (Samikshya). Urmila, too, referred to the 'widespread corruption in the government sector. In every government agency, there are middlemen. People have to access services through these middlemen'. There were 'excessive bureaucratic procedures' (Samikshya), an 'absence of institutional management . . . [and] systematic government plans to improve individual and public lives' (Ranjan), 'relying on remittance [and aid rather] than [a] self-sustained economy', 'weak provisions for service delivery' (Niharika), and 'tendency to depend on sponsored development [rather] than development initiated within' (Sujit).

Advocating for the voiceless: the case for political focus

Marginalisation as a structural issue: need for engaging in political aims and advocacy

Marginalisation was one of the major themes that participants kept returning to and provided an extensive information about it. However, the understanding of marginalisation was subjective and varied according to participants' positions informed by their self-identity – belongingness to gender, geographic reason, and ethnicity and caste groups. Marginalisation mainly meant systematic 'exclusion from, and lack of awareness of existing resources' (Urmila) and 'differential treatment based on caste, class, gender, and geography' (Niharika). It also included a 'lack of identity' (Niti) that must be viewed 'beyond poverty and caste hierarchy' (Ritesh). People's lack of access to education was an important aspect in understanding marginalisation:

> If someone does not have money, they are economically poor, a kind of marginalised population. If they have economic access, then, regardless of their low social statuses, such as caste, gender, and so forth, they are not marginalised. . . . [Even] uneducated . . . are marginalised in several ways.
>
> (Sujit)

> As a social worker, I advocate new thinking that means there is need to change the definition of marginalisation in Nepal. Marginalisation must be seen beyond poverty and caste hierarchy. There should be another framework to define marginalisation. Those who are not getting education and those who have education but they do not have opportunity are marginalised section in the society. Also, those who are motivated to contribute in the society and are not getting any support from state machinery are marginalised in the society.
>
> (Ritesh)

People were marginalised because of their caste, such as *Dalit*; access to resources, such as the landless; gender and age, such as women, children, and elderly people; geography, such as rural population; and power, such as excluded groups and minorities. From her experience of visiting 35 districts, Niti claimed that '*Dalit* are still marginal in the country'. Urmila observed,

> Those who are in the lower strata of caste are vulnerable. . . . There is wide discrimination against lower caste people . . . [and often] are excluded from utilising facilities provided by government and non-government organisations.

Marginalisation led to resource-distribution issues and stereotyping, as Niti explained: 'Those who are landless are marginal population in the country. They are chased away wherever they settle. To extent, they lack identity'. Further, 'women are treated as a second-class citizens' (Samikshya). 'They are victims of violence' (Namita). 'Rural women who are deprived of education . . . are vulnerable population. These women cannot take their life decisions, such as about marriage, reproduction, and employment. They do not have bargaining capacity' (Ranjan). 'Rural populations are marginalised in the country' (Samikshya). Sujit believed that the peoples of the Himalayas, and ethnic minorities from both Hills and Terai were powerless in mainstream of politics. Because of geographical complexities, many people in the Himalaya region could not even imagine transport facility (Ritesh). Niharika summed up the extent of marginalisation:

> Historically low caste groups are marginalised in the country. Likewise, those who have been staying in the remote areas of Himalaya, resource handicapped, excluded groups who are not represented in mainstream politics [are marginal section of the society]. Also, accessibility to resources, finance, education, and power determine

marginalisation and vulnerability. Uneducated women and children are in double marginalisation. Rural people are comparatively marginalised than those living in Kathmandu and the urban centre of the country.

Thus, participants understood the structural nature of marginalisation in Nepali society and the need to engage in macrolevel social work with a strong focus on political issues (Niharika), community (Namita), society (Samikshya), and nation (Sujit) as spaces or layers of macro practice than targeting individuals. However, the main challenge, as Sujit explained, was that social work had failed to reach beyond educational institutions to become the part of mainstream politics alongside government and non-government agencies to address the issue of marginalisation. The problem notwithstanding, Niharika suggested a political role for social work. For her, the very concept of doing social work in Nepali society involved politicking that bestowed on Nepali social workers the key role of 'becoming the voice for the voiceless'. She continued,

[It is] important to enable people to tap resources and refrain themselves from violation of their rights. Being social worker, we cannot avoid political debates. Especially Nepali society is so much related to politics . . . [social work] should focus on well-being, improved social justice, empowerment, [and] cultural awareness [of one and all].

(Niharika)

Conclusion

There are long-standing critiques against universalisation and globalisation of social work. This chapter, drawing on the ground-up evidences, synergises with those critiques and delineates how the technological transfer of social work from the 'West to the rest' has left Nepali social workers ill-prepared to respond to the Nepali socio-cultural-political contexts. More importantly, it captures Nepali social workers' critical analysis about social work education and practice as well as development-related activities. This emerging insiders' views evoke a sentiment that Nepali social workers fall in the category of 'rejectionist Global South' favouring the prospect and need for decolonisation of social work as discussed in Chapter 5. So, the next question is – how might Nepali social workers involve in incorporating their practice experiences to devise decolonised and developmental social work – which I conceptually model in the next chapter.

Decolonised and developmental Nepali social work

A model ground up

The process that began with exploring emerging social work practice in Nepal from the perspective of social workers employed in INGOs comes to an edge, in this chapter, with a model of decolonised and developmental Nepali social work. I begin this chapter with a brief summary of the participants' concerns about social work education. And then, I examine social, developmental, and political components of decolonising practice and their interplays to formulate a model of decolonised and developmental Nepali social work. In the end, I briefly discuss the model in relation to existing literatures in this area and its relevance for ongoing research and further development of socially relevant social work education and practice in Nepal.

Social workers' concerns

The participant collectively provided a critical analysis of Nepali social work education. As shown in Table 7.1, they expressed concerns about: (i) Its colonialist and imperialistic legacies that had systematically suppressed the Nepali ethos and brought a knowledge economics based on an elitist professional ideology; (ii) its urban centred concentration outside the reach of Nepal's rural poor peoples; (iii) the lack of critical interrogation of imported theories, practice frameworks, and pedagogical models; (iv) the gap between urban social work graduates and the majority rural populations oblivious to modern service and development technologies; (v) social workers' lack of will to collaborate and learn from related disciplines and theoretical discourses; (vi) the inability to develop local literature and education programs; (vii) reluctance to shift from English to local languages more comprehensible to social workers and diverse beneficiaries as the main medium of teaching; (viii) inability to move beyond professional extremism and give social work a 'vocational' ethos that better reflects the Nepali character; (ix) the absence of continued education, training, and research through which to explore education and practice models relevant to national and local contexts; (x) an inability to decide on the contextual scope and direction of social work education and practice that address contemporary Nepali social issues; (xi) lack of consideration of the development agencies, where most graduates were being employed; and (xii), above all, a failure to look back at Nepal's history, cultures, traditions, sociopolitical dynamics, government's plan, policy, and structures, and economic demands and transform social work to fit that context.

Participants were concerned about the ongoing imposition of outsiders' world views and the absence of local practice models. Outsider perspectives ignored traditionally

Table 7.1 Summary of social workers' concerns about borrowed Western social work

Bideshi nature	Lack of local base practice knowledge	Competing world views	Normative approach	Unsuitable to local developmental framework
• **Imported and imposed from outside** • **Prevailing Western theories, methods, and literature** • **Individualistic, psychologised models** • **Political economy of colonisation intended to produce cheap labour for the Western world** • **Dominance of English over local languages** • **Professional jargon and terminology hard to translate into local languages** • **Glamourised within the elitist professional club** • **Non-supportive of local social workers' 'self-expression' due to its *bideshi* nature**	• Lack of sociocultural embedded knowledge and practice models • Non-transferrable and non-communicable knowledge out of step with routinised cultural frameworks • Oblivious to Nepali social structures and cultural diversification • Lack of a critical structural perspective • Unresponsive to national and local social issues • Inability to draw on field-based practice interventions and grassroots' realities in the curriculum • Lack of a human rights perspective, advocacy, activism, and social reform ethos in education and practice	• Outsider/insider • Localisation-modernisation/westernisation • Colonialist-imperialist/sovereignty and self-determination • Long-term sustainable change/short-term rapid development • Individualism/collectivism • Linear/holistic • Knowledge economics, elitism, neoliberalist/critical, reflexive, and people-centred • Profession/vocation • Inclusion of urban elite/exclusion of rural poor • Professional extremism and elitist sectarianism/reflexive, collaborative, developmental change agents	• Becoming social worker as a continuous process rather than an end • Moral responsibility motivated by 'goodness' one could do for others • More than 'self-imposed' professional identity through association, Nepali social work should earn community sanction and credibility through its virtuous intervention designed within local boundaries • Alongside contaminating the local wisdom, social work is colonising the Nepali minds by systematically creating 'white minds in brown bodies' • The relationship is formed and valued through 'social cohesion' and 'social fabric' • Altering the concept of doing social services	• Oblivious to local development agenda, activities, and agencies • Unsuitable to reflect on local developmental tools and techniques • Its education base unable to fit itself within local development paradigm

established sociocultural knowledge systems and reflected stereotypical views of Nepali value and belief systems. Most importantly, however, given the contexts in which most graduates were employed, they lacked a critical understanding of the development frameworks and policies within which INGOs operated. Consequently, the social workers did not have the requisite skills and knowledge to work in these international development agencies.

Social components of decolonised practice

In Chapter 6, participants provided a unique understanding of Nepali society and its features. Here, in this section, I draw on from those discussions to frame the ways the social components contribute to the emerging model of decolonised and developmental social work. Contrary to missionaries' approach in the past and ongoing imperialist endeavours in the present (see Chapter 1 and Chapter 4), this section explores bottom-up how, and meanwhile why, cultural framework, centrality of local knowledge, and peoples' connection to the past history and environment and spirituality are essential in thinking about decolonised and developmental social work.

Routinised cultural framework

The findings on core components within indigenous knowledge and sociocultural systems revealed a routinised cultural framework, so-called because it was deeply embedded in Nepal's social fabric, and the collective values and norms cementing Nepali's diverse cultural and ethnic groups together. Decolonising social work, as participants claimed, required that social workers responded by focusing on 'cultural practices' (Kiran), 'cultural components' (Sujit), and 'social [and] cultural . . . dynamics' (Niharika). It would have to be responsive to the unique experiences and perspectives of Nepal's multiethnic, Indigenous Peoples 'to contribute to the betterment of the society' (Sujit). Connecting to indigenous knowledge and sociocultural systems would enable social work to firmly embed itself in long-established traditions that have sustained individual, groups, and communities for centuries.

Paropkar or charity has served Nepali's collective system well 'to respond promptly' (Niti), to find 'similarity for entry point to work with' (Ritesh), and 'to build rapport and develop trust' (Kiran) within the communities. From the participants' responses, it was clear that a decolonisation framework would be grounded in their culture, tradition, history, and family, social, and institutional ties. To some extent, the routinised cultural practices participants adhered to mirror the collective symbolic structures of people's everyday lives, their traditions and values. Participants' ability to discuss them at length showed they could explain their actions in their daily practice in terms of their cultural knowledge and values. In a sense, despite their foreign-influenced education and borrowed knowledge, they adopted an inward-looking perspective drawing on an entire set of concepts, beliefs, and perceptions about the world around them. Embracing local knowledge enabled them to understand how particular dynamics ranging from their personal life, to their daily reality and its political, socioeconomic, and cultural diversity, the institutional mechanisms, legal and policy instruments, and service approaches in the INGOs in which they worked came together as an integrated framework of local knowledge that made them aware of the 'many things happening around . . . in day-to-day life' (Samikshya). As Niti explained,

Again, we are not doing everything as informed by theoretical perspectives. Many of them come from our experience. We propagate our ideas based on the contexts. Sometimes we explain theoretical knowledge in reports but, in the practice, we work with our own perspectives. That is a different matter. . . . Mainly we are guided by our own experience. This is contradiction that we are not applying what we were taught. . . . More than theoretically informed it requires culturally sensitive skills.

Centrality of local, contextual knowledge

The participants' quest for local knowledge was nevertheless filtered through Western concepts. In other words, the social workers described the very concept of local knowledge in relation to theoretical social work knowledge borrowed from outside that did not resonate with their experiences, values, and world views. Samikshya said that her educational background had no connection to the work that she was doing:

As a student, we excessively focused on casework . . . while working in the communities we work with large groups, maybe large communities. We cannot practice casework with them. Real work is different than what we were taught . . . and that's why we need to emphasise on adoption of local knowledge, which will support Nepali social workers to work with masses.

Likewise, Niti saw local or practice contexts were different from theoretical contexts; and, thus she emphasised contextual knowledge:

The practice contexts are completely different from theoretical contexts [outsiders' construct]. I need to mobilise a mass, which requires contextual knowledge about those people. Some of theoretical knowledge only makes sense in [a] classroom.

Integrating local knowledge was seen as essential for the recognition of social work and to obtain community sanction:

If we want to contextualise social work in future, we need to relate our curriculum to our day-to-day life experience. This will make [it] easy for students to relate theoretical knowledge in the field and will also help to the recognition of social work in Nepal.

(Samikshya)

One of the participants working in the child rights sector described practice knowledge as grounded in everyday life. It was local knowledge, as Ranjan explained: 'We have to develop practice knowledge from our day-to-day lives and claim what is social work in the country'. Ritesh expanded thus:

The position where I am working now requires a lot of knowledge about society. Experience is important. Theory is just a guideline. The practice is different. Implementation is different. The implementation of theory in local context is different. For example, you cannot implement the same theoretical perspective in *badi* communities who are traditionally commercial sex workers, and in an educated community. This has not been differentiated in our education.

His insights on grounding social work interventions in local knowledge rather universal standards and principles captured the essence of decolonised social work practice in Nepal and elsewhere:

> Social work is not about formulae but a domain of context-related knowledge application. We need to analyse political, economic, cultural, and traditional dynamics of the community. When you want to assess any communities, you do not go without prior information. You analyse the community context; you conduct some research.
>
> (Ritesh)

Sujit likewise noted that 'we cannot use the same approach . . . we need to adapt . . . to changing time and society. Neither government nor any organisation has formulae procedure'. Also, in Nepal, communal conflict is masked by a thin layer of social fabric, through which violence might erupt at any moment:

> If you want to address the issue of caste discrimination, you have to keep several things in your mind. For example, if you are raising the issue of caste-based discrimination at place where there is tension between *Dalit* and non-*Dalit*, you cannot have discussion at the forum where there are Brahmin, Kshatriya, and *Dalit*. But our theory says we need to have focus group discussion where there should be four to eight group members. Sometimes social workers talk about inclusion, gender balance [as they have been defined in the West]. Applying those, can we work with the group comprising Brahmin, Kshatriya, and *Dalit*? Also, can we organise public hearing keeping *Pahade* and *Madhishe* in Terai [in the wake of emerging ethnic clashes and divisions]? There will be violence.
>
> (Ritesh)

There were elements of spontaneity in local strategies akin to what might be the art of social work. Niharika's claim of 'we have to react spontaneously' shows that local strategy is intuitive and spontaneous in nature. Possibly, it is also hard to measure and predict each specific case of local strategy used by Nepali social workers by simply using qualitative method within definite time frame. But there is link that this is the impact of broader cultural and social contexts over individual. As evidenced in participants' voices, such as 'our experience', 'our own perspective' (Niti), and 'our context' (Niharika) typically demonstrate the sources of local strategy. The marker 'our' in the source reflects participants' agreement that local strategy is informal collective contract that they apply in socially and culturally accepted manner. Informal communication, establishing some form of kinship with target groups, coordinating with experienced local staff, and identifying local strategic community leaders are most frequently used local strategies in the lives of social workers of Nepal.

> When we meet our target groups, we do not use professional approach such as setting appointments, formal introductions, telling them what our roles are. We start from informal communication. [Also] establishing relations such as of brother,

sister, uncle, aunt, father, and mother with the community people are additional benefit to work.

(Samikshya)

Likewise, to this Niti reflected,

We visit field with experienced person . . . [who] are not professionally trained social workers. . . . They know the nerves of the community affairs. They just need one clue . . . and can take up the entire conversation to maximum effective level. They are more skilful than I am. I agree social workers can make a good report based on their theoretical knowledge but working in the communities is different.

And, Ritesh explained further,

Local staffs are more knowledgeable than us. They know who to approach. They have clear ideas of localities. Our community facilitators communicate with target groups. Our facilitators encourage community people to attend community meetings. They use local and informal approaches, which is very effective.

All knowledge, even local knowledge, had to be adapted to changing needs and problems: 'We need to adopt changing time and society' (Sujit). Importantly, local knowledge was culturally sensitive reflecting the unique cultural and spiritual identity of Nepali communities, which were often grounded in experience, observation, and self-reflection: 'General knowledge and common sense' (Kiran), 'life experience' (Samikshya), 'culture', and 'interaction with people from different walks of lives' (Sujit).

In the context of applying their social work knowledge in the field, participants talked about adopting alternative knowledge, using an informal approach, and responding spontaneously to embedded sociocultural norms and practices. They highlighted the importance of direct experience, observation, and self-reflection as a knowledge source. Of necessity, traditional cultural practices were central to appropriate social work knowledge and traditional belief systems had to be accommodated. Citing the example of 'norms and values of [Nepali] places' as integral parts of traditional dynamic, Kiran, a social worker born and brought up in rural part of Nepal, emphasised the integration of culture in social work practice:

I come from a rural area and I know about the [traditional and cultural] dynamics of that place. I have observed them and have learnt many things about rural areas through my experiences and self-reflections. I think this aspect should be integrated in social work trainings. Social work education needs to bring knowledge from there. The norms and values of those places must be known to social work educators and taught to future generations of social workers.

For him, the concepts of rapport building, acceptance, and non-judgemental attitude taught within social work education programs are implicit norms in traditional Nepali society, which did not require Western standardisation and interpretation:

We might have used tools and techniques such as rapport building and social work principles. But, I am surprised if those tools and techniques should be part of syllabus . . . we learn about rapport building and acceptance, non-judgemental attitude since our childhood. These are core to our culture.

(Kiran)

Connecting to the past

A component of decolonising social work found in the literature but scarcely mentioned by the participants was an awareness of historical trauma and connecting with the past to move forward into the future. There were some exceptions, however. Sujit referred to the process of understanding, reflecting, and applying the historically developed community development experiences, approaches, and contextual knowledge, including past stories:

> Look at your own back . . . let's look back to our history and craft social work [accordingly]. . . . [It] has lot to contribute to the development of Nepali model of social work . . . we need to look back to our history [to understand] what our ancestors have done for community development. . . . We can look back to our pasts and see how stories, community development experiences, approaches, including social work approaches have been developed.

(Sujit)

Nevertheless, there were many ways in which history and tradition played through the daily lives of Nepali peoples, and in which knowledge handed down through the generations knitted together the social fabric creating strong familial and community connections.

Strong environmental and spiritual connections

Ranjan referred to 'our unique livelihood strategy' by which he meant the deep connection with the environment within Nepali peoples' tradition and rituals; Nepali people treat nature as a god. In times of crisis, their veneration for nature has proven to be a great support and helped them to control overwhelming emotions like fear. Such natural healing practices had to be integrated into decolonising social work interventions. As Ranjan explained, Nepali people are deeply connected to the land and live close to nature and this is an intrinsic part of their spirituality. This underlies communal solidarity:

> In terms of strength, we have our own unique livelihood strategies. Maybe we can say it is our traditional practices. For instance, during dozens of aftershocks [on April and May 2015] people were overwhelmed of anxious, hopeless, and fear. To overcome distress anxiety and feelings, they gathered together and carried out *Bhumi Puja* and *Kshama Puja*. Nepali people consider nature as god. Through these rituals, they reflected whether they have done any mistakes; whether they have angered mother nature. These rituals help people to control emotions and fears. Probably many foreign relief providers who came to Nepal that time did not understand these local livelihood strategies. Nepal is [a] faith-based society where they consider nature a god. We should design social work considering traditional beliefs, responses, and ways of life. We need to explore logics in those practices. Also, we need to explore how those practices are going to help people in true sense.

Developmental components of decolonising practice

Given both *bideshi vikash* and *swadeshi aadhar* were part of the problem than solution, participants viewed decolonising social work as an opportunity to integrate people-centred, bottom-up development in Nepali social work. The social characteristics, social problems, and issues for Nepali social work mentioned in Chapter 2 and Chapter 3 as well as explored in the previous chapter related mainly to poverty-related discrimination and oppression of minorities, landlessness, and gender-related violence. Relatedly, this section explains the developmental goals of Nepali social work.

People-centred developmental focus

To a greater extent, participants emphasised that Nepali social workers should have knowledge of, and adhere to, the people-centred development process. They also viewed building collaboration with development stakeholders, including GOs, NGOs, and local formal and informal agencies, as essential strategies to ignite 'social movement' (Kiran), 'social change', and 'conne[cting] community with government's policies and programs' (Namita). Within its people-centred developmental ambit, the major themes concerned to:

- 'Engage local peoples in development plan and policies' (Kiran).
- Embrace 'culturally sensitive', 'community focused' (Niti), and 'social responsive' (Niharika) approaches to 'make community independent' (Niti).
- 'Emphasise on capacity development of community' (Niharika).
- 'Focus on [maximising] welfare and economic benefits' (Sujit) for people.

In other words, Sujit suggested that social work should 'contribute to community development, economic benefit, and upliftment of marginalised population' (Sujit). It was this developmental focus currently missing in decolonising discourse that added a new dimension to what decolonised social work in Nepal might entail, hence the move to developmental, decolonising practice. Of necessity, to achieve this involved balancing internal – academic institutions, social work educators, and social work graduates – and external forces – government and INGOs. The collectively identified certain key goals that might accomplish this are illustrated in Table 7.2.

Likewise, Namita and Ritesh talked about how their experiences in development agency had redefined and reshaped their practice knowledge. Namita said, 'We learn in the agencies. Everyone . . . faces a lot of problems [in the beginning where they are employed] . . . that is the only way if one wants to survive [in the agency]'. Similarly, Ritesh stated, 'We come to know about . . . [practising social work] through our work [and] practical experiences'. Niharika clearly understood that 'job market for [social workers] is competitive. All social workers cannot sustain in the organisation' unless they learn anew. Samikshya noted the large part her experience had played in practicing development:

[These are] life experiences that enrich my work. It is like seeing-learning-doing. Our culture, tradition, socialisation, norms, and values have great impacts on our work. But, the source of social work's knowledge . . . has not come from what I mentioned just now. . . . [If we adopt them firmly] we will have maximum benefit.

Table 7.2 Balancing internal and external forces

Internal forces			External forces	
Academic institutions	Social work educators	Social work practitioners/graduates	Government	INGOs
• **Give social work education the same priority as other disciplines** • **Move beyond treating social work education as a business** • **Emphasise the development of a context-responsive social work curriculum** • **Fight for the recognition of social work in Nepal** • **Engage practitioners in teaching** • **Focus on quality social work graduates** • **Coordinate with and receive feedback from INGOs**	• Be qualified to teach and well informed about local debates • Inculcate the value of localisation and contextualisation of social work among • See the importance of development and development-related content in the curriculum	• Organise and collectively discuss the future of social work • Make government feel their presence by partnering in government-initiated development plans and activities • Work toward creating a context suitable social work policy, which has been missing until now	• Engage social workers in its various structures • Recognise social work • Monitor social work institutions and social work graduates • Create space for social work graduates in its line ministries relevant to social work • Sponsor and encourage social work institutions to design social work to be responsive to the Nepali context • Create jobs for social work graduates	• Recognise social work graduates and employ them in social work posts • Provide feedback on the effectiveness of social work in development fields • Be aware social work institutes and graduates where social work exactly fits in their organisation • Put pressure on social work education institutions to teach development-related content

Familial, societal, and agency networks fashioned 'self-consciousness' (Kiran), 'life-experience' (Samikshya), 'long-term engagement' (Ritesh), and developing 'own perspective' (Niti). Ritesh observed that 'experience is [an] important' aspect of social work practice. Thus, decolonising social work should be anchored in first-hand experiences and work from the ground up keeping people in the centre of developmental activities. It only emerges through practitioners' continuous engagement with the people they serve.

Self-reliance based community development focus

Social workers had to emphasise building and strengthening 'self-reliance' – an approach that encouraged 'self-sufficiency' and 'self-empowerment', Sujit noted. It was equally important for participants that the process of community development included Nepal's diverse peoples and a respect for differences based on caste, ethnicity, language, and culture. This led them to envision social work as 'flexible' (Sujit) with 'its boundary . . . remain[ing] open' (Ritesh) to update social work as Nepali society evolves in the time continuum.

Livelihood strategy emerged as a strong theme for promoting self-reliance within the community development approach. For example, Urmila actively taught and prepared local women's groups in a way to use their livelihood strategy 'to address their problems by themselves'. This way, she believed that women's groups could use their 'knowledge and skills . . . [to] access government and other resources' even after professional support terminated. Sujit also referred to livelihood strategies as the important aspects for promoting self-reliance for the local community peoples:

> Simply saying I have bachelor or master degree in social work and critically applying them in the field are two different things. We need to develop our understanding from those theories. We should develop our social work in a way that it matches peoples' day-to-day capacity and livelihood strategies. . . . We need to customise Western social work according to our peoples' capacity . . . apply them in the ways that peoples do not rely on social workers' support in long run.

Peace and security oriented safety focus

Developmental components also related to safety focus and the importance of peace and security. According to participants, there was need to promote a 'philosophy of safer life' (Ritesh) by 'maximising . . . [peoples'] participation in development and governance considering issues of social justice' (Ranjan). Thus, Ritesh linked 'feeling safe' and its several dimensions with social work:

> The main focus of social work must be community security a safe society, then a safe nation. . . . I can say, social work must intend to create safer community, safer society, and safer nation . . . guided by philosophy of safer life . . . [Feeling safe] should be our common future. . . . Security is related with human rights. Everyone must enjoy his or her rights. Everyone has right to live safe. . . . It is also people's responsibility to take initiations toward creating safer community and safe life.

For Niharika, the right to peace was 'directly associated with political actions, such as empowerment, capacity building, and sensitization . . . the matters of political and civil rights are required to enable peoples' safety'. She further claimed that the right to peace would ensure Nepali people's 'well-being and will improve social justice' (Niharika). Nevertheless, feeling safe went beyond the mere notion of rights and justice to include:

- 'Social capital' (Kiran) and 'empowerment' (Namita).
- 'Education and awareness' (Namita).
- 'Freedom and upliftment of oppressed peoples' (Namita).
- 'Economic reforms by engaging poor in income-generation programs' (Urmila).
- 'Policy enhancement emphasising people-centred social policies' (Namita).
- 'Building civil society through greater participation of people in governance' (Ranjan).

Participants broader understanding of feeling safe signalled a strong focus on rights-based social work practice with its emancipatory goals that I discuss in subsequent section.

Political components of decolonising practice

Solutions to marginalisation lay in political focus by educating people (Samikshya, Ritesh, and Sujit), 'raising awareness' (Namita), 'empowering and capacity building' (Samikshya), 'collaborating the efforts of government organisations, non-government organisations, and political parties' (Ranjan), 'improving the economic statuses' (Sujit), taking 'actions . . . within the cultural frame of reference . . . [to avoid] . . . conflict' (Samikshya), 'strengthening existing rules, laws, and policies' (Namita), 'enhancing capacity of people' (Samikshya), and 'making government services equitably accessible and approachable' (Tulshi). The participants envisioned that the issues of marginalisation could be addressed using rights-based social work with strong political goals aimed at advocating for the voiceless by:

- Integrating rights-aligned discourse into practice.
- Framing political, anti-oppressive practice approaches.
- Engaging in transformative action.
- Emphasising on policy and development.

Integrating rights-aligned discourse into practice

The participants acknowledged the need for translating the rights-aligned discourse such as *samajik nyay* (Ranjan) and *samanta* (Niti), the protection of human rights and promotion of social justice and equality in other words, into practice to address the issues of marginalisation in Nepali society. As Niti explained,

> Gradually the demand for social work is increasing in NGOs and INGOs of the country. If social workers can engage them in activism certainly they will be recognised in the country. We have a lot to contribute. . . . Now, as I see, the main role of social workers is activism because all issues are structural and connected

with rights, justice, and fair treatment. Rights-based approach should inform the ideal of social work.

Framing political, anti-oppressive practice approaches

According to Sujit, political, anti-oppressive approaches were necessary to uplift the status of Nepali marginalised and vulnerable populations. Likewise, Samikshya believed that political, anti-oppressive focus of social work would '. . . help those who . . . [were] dominated and oppressed in the societies . . . [and using them as practice approaches would] uplift the bottom section of the society'. To this, Niharika recommended,

> It is important for social workers to understand the ways power and politics significantly yield marginalised population in our society. For example, the subordinated status of *Dalits, Madheshis,* and *Janajatis* in our society is so much related to the discourse of power and politics. . . . [Hence,] . . . being social workers there is need that we frame the issues of marginalisation within political understanding and use the right intervention [that is political, anti-oppressive practice approach] to address these.

However, Namita raised concerns about,

> What is social action, how to deal with peoples' [political issues] were not taught. [Also] we do not have ideas of petitions, protest, and other activities that are frequently occurring in the country. . . . There should be more focus on political issues [and] government rules. Political education should be emphasised.

Engaging in transformative action

The political components of decolonising practice also emphasised transformative action meaning engaging Nepali peoples in systematic programs of change for socioeconomic 'empowerment' (Namita), 'income-generation activities' (Urmila), and 'labour-retention' programs (Sujit). Namita observed that women were

> suffering from violence, [mainly] domestic violence. First, we need to aware them. . . . Usually, women do not know about rules and laws about our country. We can provide information about rules and laws to those women. . . . The main aim of social work [while working in the women sector] is empowerment.
>
> (Namita)

Likewise, Urmila highlighted on the need for income generation program: 'Social work should target the population who are under developed. . . . Since most of the people are poor in the country, social worker should be also engaged in income-generation program'. Participants also observed the need for social workers' engagement in fostering innovation and entrepreneurship to retain Nepali labour force at home (Sujit and Urmila). Samikshya summed up this saying, 'An empowered, aware, and economically sound person can enhance self-image and lead a better quality of life in the society'.

Emphasising policy and development

Namita believed that Nepali peoples' orientation about and engagement with government policies was not satisfactory. She claimed that social workers could become a link between the people and government: 'There is greater need of social workers in our context so that people can be connected with the policies of the government'. Nevertheless, she raised concerns:

> Where is Nepal related laws and policies? What are government's policy measures and development frameworks that should be reflected in our educational contents and practice interventions.
>
> (Namita)

Similarly, Ranjan illustrated how social work can engage into policy-related activities for social change process especially in the child rights sector:

> Mainly we address child-related violence. Many of child-related violence are traditionally accepted. Our organisation mainly works to address five thematic areas – child marriage, corporal punishment, sexual abuse and exploitation, child trafficking, and child labour. We seek to address these problems at macrolevel. Therefore, our main agenda is to help government to formulate necessary programs and policy to address child related issues.

Model of decolonised and developmental Nepali social work practice

Drawing on participants' concerns and visions, now I present the model of decolonised and developmental Nepali social work. Gregor (2006) believed that theoretical models 'are practical because they allow knowledge to be accumulated in a systematic manner and this accumulated knowledge enlightens professional practice' (p. 613). A theoretical model not only answers 'what is' but also seeks to explain 'why it is so'. 'A useful theory is one that tells an enlightening story about some phenomenon. It is a story that gives . . . [us] new insights and broadens . . . [our] understanding of the phenomenon' (Anfara & Mertz, 2006, p. xvii) 'as means for understanding our world' (Castells, 2000, p. 390). It is important to reiterate that from the outset the aim of this book was to address what decolonised and developmental social work might entail by examining Nepali sociopolitical realities. The model of social work presented herein rests on internally driven knowledge frameworks with strong grounding in Nepali sociocultural traditions. Knowledge about local contexts and cultures, Nepali history, and the factors that have shaped the contemporary social and political landscape is essential to complement understanding of human behaviour given social work's pivotal focus on human interaction in response to the broader sociocultural, economic, and political environment. A holistic understanding is pivotal to socially responsive, culturally sensitive social work practice not only for bringing desired changes in peoples' lives but also for binding them together in solidarity to view future meaningful and hopeful. This section discusses the theoretical underpinnings for the model relating to its core foci – cultural, structural, contextual, and developmental, as shown in Figure 7.1.

The model of decolonised and developmental social work practice in Nepal, once implemented and used to inform curriculum change, will lead to the 'Nepalisation' of social work because of its grounding in contextual experience and its culturally

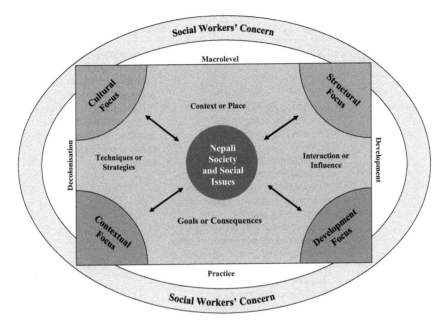

Figure 7.1 Model of decolonised and developmental Nepali social work

and socially responsive nature. On the one hand, this model involved uncovering the colonial sentiments embedded in borrowed Western social work knowledge and, on the other, examining what was unique to Nepal, and bringing a heretofore unexplored 'developmental' perspective to decolonising practice, as discussed above in this chapter. The purpose was to dissociate Nepali social work from the ongoing hegemonic, colonial, and neoliberal bent of imported social work. The model presented in Figure 7.1 draws on aspects of imported social work education and practice that are worth retaining, such as strategies for the development of cultural competence, and seeks to restore the 'social' in Nepali social work through its people first, community focus. As shown in Table 7.3, the model is:

- Responsive to Nepali sociocultural traditions, that is, cultural focus.
- Responsive to power and structure, that is, structural focus.
- Responsive to local problems and issues, that is, contextual focus.
- Responsive to poverty, that is, developmental focus.

Cultural focus: responsive to Nepali sociocultural traditions

A major premise of decolonisation theory relates to cultural appropriateness, that is, responsiveness to local/national sociocultural conditions. This relates to social work theory on cultural and ethnic sensitivity, diversity, and indigenisation. At the centre of

Table 7.3 Focus of decolonised and developmental Nepali social work

Focus	Strategies	Assumptions
Cultural	• Culturally sensitive practice	• A culturally sensitive social work strengthens insider perspectives within the practice
Structural	• Furthering rights and justice concerns by engaging in empowering, transformative action • Developing political, anti-oppressive approaches to bring marginalised groups into decision-making structures and processes • Transforming peoples' socioeconomic status through empowerment, awareness, income generation, and labour-retention programs • Focusing on policy and development by gaining entry in government's development planning and policy execution processes	• A rights-based, social justice perspective will alter the distribution of power and create a more inclusive society
Contextual	• Customising and fitting imported development strategies • Making knowledge comprehensible and suitable to local community groups	• Contextualisation accommodates local world views and responds to day to day social issues
Developmental	• Community development • Putting people first • Social movements for social change • Building and strengthening community self-reliance • Inclusive development • Multiple stakeholder engagement • Socially responsive, community-focused capacity building drawing on first-hand experiences and local knowledge • Building peace and security by promoting local strategies to minimise conflict • Livelihood strategies to encourage self-reliance • Using government and local resources	• Grassroots bottom-up development strengthens local peoples' participation and decision-making capabilities in development • Community development responds to unique identities and local needs, and encourages community ownership of development • Safety is a need and right. Participation in peacebuilding initiatives will establish a safe society and, thus, a safer life for all • This will address Nepal's overriding issue of poverty through improved community engagement in income-generating activities and livelihood-sustaining strategies

the model is Nepali society and social issues, that is, the context to which the decolonised model seeks to respond.

As participants revealed above and also discussed in Chapter 2, Nepali society stands at the crossroad of its enduring, traditional past and gradually evolving, modern worldview. The participants valued deep-rooted Nepali sociocultural traditions. They saw these as the ties binding Nepal's cohesive social fabric together. Traditional values created a normative dynamic that was historically and culturally embedded within the institutions of Nepali society and its structural diversification. Traditional social norms guide, control, regulate, and dominate Nepali peoples' social and interpersonal interactions. Paradoxically, Nepali peoples' sense of membership, belonging, solidarity, and identity have been consciously or deliberately built around deep-seated status differences, such as ascribed association into caste and ethnic groups, as well as linguistic, cultural, and regional affiliations. Inter-group differences, that is, differences between members of different social groups have been socially and culturally accepted and managed. Despite these differences, 'collective experience', 'collective consciousness', 'collective wisdom', and 'collective action' are celebrated and form the social glue that brings people together when they need to work cooperatively, such as in times of natural disasters. Participant's narratives carried the symbolic significance of a 'we feeling' – collectiveness, feelings of community, and mutual interdependence, of helping one another, unity, solidarity, and togetherness.

The dominance of contextual and local values distinguishes Nepali society from the individualism, modernism (or post-modernism), and industrialism (or post-industrialism) of the Western nation states from which its imported social work knowledge comes. These values forced the participants to examine their borrowed social work knowledge and practice models to free them from the grip of its imperialist and colonialist leanings, and make them fit into Nepal's unique sociocultural and political context. What thus emerged was a form of localised, decolonised Nepali social work that recognised that individual identities were shaped by broader familial, social, and cultural interactions and unique practices. These comprised rituals, festivals, and established traditional norms, such as *guthi, dharma*, and *paropkar* or *sewa* that gave a collective meaning to notions of the individual 'self'. Samikshya conveyed this sense of collective identity when she claimed that 'what she is today and how she reacts as a social worker in a community setting is the influence of her family and surrounding environment'.

Essentially, then decolonised and developmental social work practice seeks to respond to the uniqueness of Nepali society and traditional cultural norms and values alien to Western cultures. The Western notion of universal human rights is compatible with the collective solidarity of in-group relationships but is unlikely to transcend deep-seated caste and class divisions. Rather than a capacity for individual freedom, collective rights are linked to duties and responsibilities that are deeply embedded in Nepali traditions. Kiran and Ranjan provided examples in relation to corporal punishment and divorce respectively in the previous chapter.

In Nepal's multilayered, highly stratified, and culturally diverse society, a cohesive social space is produced by the normative dynamics of everyday life. Pressures of time are foreign to Nepali people, who prefer to do things slowly. Gradual development, growth, or progress is favoured and setbacks optimistically approached as temporary and surmountable. Modernisation requires an openness to change not readily embraced within strongly bounded cultures and traditional norms that have enabled people to survive for centuries. Thus, decolonised and developmental social work builds on the strengths of local communities and the cooperative sociocultural values that have long-sustained them. It is embedded in routinised cultural practices and the collective symbolic structures of people's everyday lives.

Structural focus: responsive to power and structure

The structural focus is underpinned by social and political theories about the way in which social structures and policies entrench disadvantage and oppression, and the intersectionalities of age, ethnicity, caste, and gender. This goes beyond an understanding of the factual characteristics of Nepali society and the nature and source of social problems to a critical analysis of the factors that oppress *Dalits*, Janajatis, Madheshis, Muslims, and other vulnerable groups such as women and children. A structural focus is undergirded by theories of human rights and social justice, and anti-oppressive and anti-racist practice.

The deeply rooted social issues and resultant structural inequalities based on caste, ethnicity, class, gender, age, geography, and resource centralisation require such a macrolevel, structural response that acknowledge the way power and unequal social relations lead to the systematic marginalisation of minority and caste and ethnic groups. Poverty, discrimination, and oppression characterise the lives of these groups, who lack access to education, land, and development. In the absence of a rights culture, discrimination against women persists. The most excluded groups in Nepali society are deeply affected by political instability and environmental disasters.

Structural interactions in Nepali society lead to the ongoing marginalisation, discrimination, and oppression of vulnerable groups that endure economic hardship and gross social injustices. Hence, the structural focus of decolonised and development social work seeks to eliminate social disadvantage and oppression maintained by intra- and inter-group differences. Furthermore, it envisions social workers' political roles and macrolevel interventions and strategies to promote human well-being, social justice, empowerment, and acceptance of diversity. It seeks structural change to alter the institutional bases of oppressive power relations and unequal access to resources. It seeks to empower disadvantage groups to gain greater access to socioeconomic opportunities and political decision-making.

Contextual focus: responsive to local problems and issues

Theories of indigenisation and decolonisation underpin the contextual focus by relating to the importance of fit between social work and the context in which it is practised, in this case, the Nepali social, economic, cultural, and political context and the extant policies and social service structures and service-delivery mechanisms. The theory of indigenisation deems home-grown social work preferable to borrowed – colonialist and imperialist – Western social work and practice, which is enriched by local knowledge that enhances social workers' capacity to resist colonising forces and devise transformative, emancipatory practice responses that are people-centred and address sociostructural problems. Such practice suggests a shift from individualised microlevel casework to socially responsive macrolevel social work interventions.

A key issue identified by the participants was discrimination and oppression of minorities, landlessness, gender-related violence, trafficking of girls, exploitation and abuse of children through child labour practices, use of violence, and corporal punishment, children living on the streets, and elder care. These were issues they had encountered in their respective INGOs, which were not necessarily addressed in their social work education. Most INGOs worked from a human rights framework and a development paradigm that sought community self-reliance. However, paradoxically, they engendered dependency since community projects could not survive without foreign aid.

Nepali social problems were described as complex, interconnected, and deeply rooted in the country's sociocultural traditions. Solutions advanced included stronger policies, education, and capacity building, and making government-provided services accessible. Social workers were seen to have a role in linking people to services and engaging in community development projects to reduce *inter alia* landlessness, child-related exploitation, the isolation of elderly people, gender-related violence, early girl marriage, and *Chhaupadi Pratha*. These complex problems are rooted in patriarchal social relations that disadvantage women and girls who are more likely to experience economic deprivation and have little decision-making power in the family. Poverty was an overriding issue depriving people of education and limiting job opportunities. Many were forced to migrate to countries in the Middle East and Malaysia in the Southeast Asia in search of work. Many families depended on remittances from family members working abroad.

Developmental focus: responsive to poverty

The contextual focus emphasises cultural appropriateness and structural interventions that lead to development-focused approaches to address poverty and inequality. The theoretical premise of this developmental focus is that decolonised and developmental social work simultaneously engages with development agencies already applying rights-based development processes and focuses on broader structural problems sustaining poverty and inequality, and disadvantaging some social groups. It suggests macrolevel interventions, such as community development. Relevant here is the theory on community assets, strengths, capacity building, participation, and empowerment. The theory of community development stresses strategies that enhance bottom-up, grassroots engagement, mutual interdependence, cooperation, and community self-reliance and self-determination, and give people the right to decide their own needs and priorities. It stresses participatory, people-centred, community-based strategies aimed at developing sustainable livelihoods and income-generating programs, and engages local agencies and multiple stakeholders in solidarity through participatory development strategies.

Given Nepal's history of conflict and political instability, building a safe society through peaceful means to enable people to be free from fear and want is an important aspect of community development. Sustainable livelihoods depend on peace and security, and income-generating opportunities within local communities, especially given the geographical complexities of the country.

The analyses showed that imported or borrowed social work was unable to respond to the development needs of local communities and critically manage structural issues embedded in Nepal's social, cultural, and political interactions or empower people to participate in their own development or engage in political activism and enhance their representation in government structures and non-government agencies. What is needed is people-centred sustainable economic growth and social development. The model is developmental in the sense that it is grounded in:

• An understanding of Nepal's socioeconomic dependency on an external international development paradigm and recognition of its counter effects.
• A critical analysis of the government's failure to govern due to political instability, deep-rooted corruption, nepotism, and favouritism, weak policies and their implementation, over regulation and red tape, inefficient and ineffective public sector management, and inability to finance development initiatives without foreign assistance.
• The view that an inclusive 'New Nepal' needs to shift gradually toward greater self-sufficiency and self-reliance.

Developmental social work requires an epistemological and technological shift in focus from individualistic and psychologised practice frameworks to community focused, socially responsive, developmental practice to uplift Nepal's many marginalised and oppressed populations. Participants believed that Nepali social work must embark on inclusive, insider-initiated, bottom-up grassroots community development to ensure self-determination and local ownership of development initiatives. Given Nepal's stormy, conflict-ridden political instability, 'feeling safe' emerged as an important priority for Nepali social workers.

Developmental methods include community-led development, community organisation, assets-, needs-based, and culturally sensitive approaches, capacity-or strengths-focused development building on social capital and empowerment, education, and awareness. Within the developmental method, social workers also emphasise on freedom and upliftment of oppressed peoples, economic reforms by engaging poor in income generation programs, people-centred social policies, and building civil society through greater participation of people in local governance.

Implications in social work: synergies with extant literature

The development of mainstream social work and its *aides-de-camp*, global social work, universal social work, international social work, and cross-cultural social work have been strongly critiqued for their hegemonic, imperialistic, and colonising agendas. Following decades of criticism, the idea of decolonising social work, with its explicit advocacy for the right to local self-determination, is taking shape. In this book, I have developed a home-grown model grounded in the daily life experiences of Nepali social workers. It promises to contribute to the decolonisation movement in social work not only through its empirical grounding but also through its insider's point of view in Nepal. Having described the components and focus of the model, it is also important to examine how it coheres with the extant literature (see Table 7.4).

Mainstream social work has been contested in Africa, Asia, Australia, Canada, and the USA for its imperialist, colonialist, and expansionist nature (Hetherington, 2009; Midgley, 1981; Sinclair, 2004; Yip, 2005a; Weaver, 1999). Long-standing struggles for culturally sensitive and socially responsive social work were, by and large, rooted in Jane Adam's idea of community development (Adams, 1910; Lundblad, 1995). The increasing focus on professionalisation led social work to abandon its 'social' mission to

Table 7.4 Integration with extant literature

Key focus	Extant literature
Indigenisation	Berking (1996), Canda (1988), Canda and Furman (1999), Coates et al. (2006), Gilligun and Furness (2005), Gray et al. (2008), Strug (2006), Weaver (1999)
Locally and culturally relevant knowledge and practice frameworks	Bruyere (1999), Gray, Coates, Yellow Bird, and Hetherington (2013b), Green (1982, 1999), Hardcastle et al. (1997), Hurdle (2002), Hetherington (2009), Lum (1999), Midgley (1981, 2008), Nagpaul (1972), Nimmagadda and Cowger (1999), Ragab (1982, 1990), Pinderhuges (1984), Shawky (1972), Yip (2005a)
Context focused and responsive to address macrolevel structural social issues	Bricker-Jenkins et al. (1991), Ferguson (2002), Gray and Webb (2013a), Gray (2005), Dominelli (1997), Mullaly (2009), Powell (2001), Schlesinger and Devore (1995), Specht and Courtney (1994), Walton and Nasr (1988)
Development-related activities	Healy and Link (2012), Ife (1995, 2013), Kenny (2010), Patel and Hochfeld (2012)
Social work and social development	Butterfield and Tasse (2013), Elliot (1993), Gray (2002), Hugman (2016), Midgley (2014), Midgley and Conley (2010)

serve society, especially the poor and oppressed (Specht & Courtney, 1994). The move to private practice puts social work further along the path of therapeutic individualism and aligned it with right-wing, neoconservative politics, as Hardcastle, Wenocur, and Powers (1997) observed:

> The problem is not so much that individual social workers have abandoned the traditional mission of the profession and, in a sense, the profession, but rather that the profession itself has abandoned its historic mission, the community, and the community's most needy and vulnerable citizens.
>
> (p. 9)

Indigenisation became a central concern in 1972 when Shawky raised questions about the fit between imported (Western) social work and local needs and contexts. Structural social work (Mullaly, 2009), feminist social work (Bricker-Jenkins, Hooyman, & Gottlieb, 1991), anti-racist social work (Dominelli, 1997), and critical social work (Allan, Briskman, & Pease, 2009; Gray & Webb, 2013a, 2013b) have all highlighted how social structures maintain social injustice and the dominance of hegemonic Western world views that privilege certain groups and disadvantage others. This discourse was extended by decolonisation scholars who have critiqued the colonising and oppressive tendencies of Western social work (Hardcastle et al., 1997; Specht & Courtney, 1994); its universal and global strategic aspirations (Gray, 2005; Yip, 2005a); and imperialistic and territorialising world views (Coates, Gray, & Hetherington, 2006; Gray, Yellow Bird, & Coates, 2008; Midgley, 1981, 2008; Weaver, 1999). Many scholars have critiqued processes that enforce Western social work in non-Western contexts like Nepal (Gray, Coates, Yellow Bird, & Hetherington, 2013c; Nagpaul, 1972; Sinclair, 2004; Specht & Courtney, 1994; Tamburro, 2013; Waterfall, 2002) and highlight the need to embrace locally sensitive and contextual-informed practice knowledge and skills to serve the society where it is positioned (Gray, Coates, & Yellow Bird, 2008a; Powell, 2001).

As shown in Table 7.4, these scholars have centred their arguments variously on:

- Culturally sensitivity, culturally appropriateness, cultural competence, cultural awareness, cultural relevance, and culturally embedded and culturally safe social work.

  (Green, 1982, 1999; Hurdle, 2002; Lum, 1999; Pinderhuges, 1979, 1984; Schlesinger & Devore, 1995; Weaver, 1999)

- Structural, anti-oppressive, and anti-racist social work practice.

  (Baines, 2011; Dominelli, 1998; Ferguson, 2002; Sinclair & Albert, 2008)

- Developmental social work, social development, and community development.

  (Butterfield & Tasse, 2013; Gray, 2002; Healy & Link, 2012; Hugman, 2016; Midgley & Conley, 2010; Patel & Hochfeld, 2012)

- Contextualisation and authentisation of locally responsive social work.

  (Gray et al., 2008a; Nimmagadda & Cowger, 1999; Ragab, 1982, 1990; Walton & Nasr, 1988)

- Decolonisation.

  (Bruyere, 1999; Gray et al., 2013c; Tamburro, 2013; Yellow Bird, 2008)

These authors have argued for the development of situated and contextual knowledge responsive to local contexts. They are clear in their standpoint that the legitimatisation and social sanctioning of social work in local contexts is only possible when professional knowledge, values, and skills are responsive to local issues and practitioners are accountable to local communities.

Similar arguments are evident in the literature on social and community development (Ife, 1995, 2013; Kenny, 2010; Netting, Kettner, & McMurtry, 2004). Ife (1995, 2013) stressed the importance of community development and claimed social workers' roles and skills in relation to community development were fluid and contingent. Gray (2002) suggested that developmental social work emphasised community strengths and capacity building in bringing about desirable change in the lives of local communities. Patel (2005) highlighted the need for development policies and structures, noting problems in policy formulation and implementation, and inefficient public sector management were root causes of development failure in South Africa. Further, Patel (2005) saw the importance of social development practices and policies to 'meet needs, promote rights, manage social problems, and facilitate the maximisation of opportunities to achieve social well-being and the promotion of human empowerment and social inclusion' (p. 203). Midgley (2014) defined social development as 'a process of planned social change designed to promote the well-being of a population as a whole within the context of dynamic and multifaceted development process' (p. 13).

Both developmental and decolonising social work have emerged in recent decades as distinctly defined approaches to social work in the Global South or within non-Western groups in the Global North. Yet, both approaches remain marginal to mainstream social work practice. The decolonising social work literature has focused largely on the indigenisation discourse using illustrative cases from non-Western and indigenous contexts where there is

> acknowledgement and incorporation of the strengths of Indigenous communities . . . to protect and restore Indigenous territories, natural resources, sacred sites, languages, cultures, beliefs, values, relationships, system of governance, intellectual property and self-determination.
>
> (Gray et al., 2013b, p. 7)

Thus, wittingly or unwittingly, it has overlooked the composition of societies like Nepal where more than indigeneity, ethnicity, caste, and geography are the basis of marginalisation. Therefore, more than indigeneity, it is decolonising approach required for social work in Nepal. On the other hand, while the developmental focus in social work addresses the need for development, it has given little critical attention within its discourse to the colonial nature of development itself, which was imposed on non-Western contexts like Nepal. While promoting the narrative of 'self-sufficiency', it has overlooked the role of developmental agencies – both international and national – in promoting neoliberalism and dependency-oriented Western development like Nepal. Thus, the decolonising and developmental social work literature has yet to address critical questions relating to its implications for underdeveloped nations like Nepal. How does decolonising and developmental social work engender emancipatory goals of human rights and social justice? How do they promote self-determination (in decolonising sense) and human well-being (in development sense)? How do they overcome the dominant dependency-generating development model? These questions can be better answered by examining the relationship between decolonising and developmental social work since both have the same goals. This book offers an interpretation of decolonised and developmental social work that might address the complex, interrelated, structural, and social issues of Nepal. It suggests that decolonised and developmental social work best reflects emerging practice. It responds to social workers' desire to exercise their autonomy and develop Nepali models appropriate to local sociopolitical realities; promotes community 'self-reliance' and puts people first; gives social workers a structural focus to critique social policy and services structures and externally imposed, dependency-driven development frameworks; promotes anti-oppressive, rights-based, inclusive developmental practice and macrolevel interventions; and marks a new beginning for Nepali social work that empowers social workers to gain the sanction of grassroots communities. The model calls on social workers to address poverty; eliminate injustices against caste and ethnic groups, women, children, and minorities; practice community development; and participate in policymaking.

Conclusion

Drawing on the perspective and experience of the Nepali social workers employed in INGOs, this chapter has presented a ground-up model of decolonised and developmental Nepali social work. In so doing, it acknowledges that shifting the ground of social work from Western influenced worldview to Nepali model not only is about equipping Nepali social workers with self-determination but also is essential given the unique features of Nepali society that distinguish it from Western society and the complex, macrolevel social issues to which Nepali social workers are attempting to respond. Importantly, the critical, emancipatory, and both post-colonial and post-developmental natures of the model advocate that the integration of locally relevant knowledge in social work is people-centred and empowerment oriented that encourage self-help, self-reliance, and self-determination to build sustainable social work in Nepal.

Chapter 8

Moving forward

With the introduction of the model of decolonised and developmental social work and its interpretations and focus, this book has come to conclusion in this chapter. The process started with the critical concerns relating to colonial and imperial roots of social work in Nepal. Within the grounded theory tradition, it not only critically explored social work practice in relation to broader Nepali social, economic, cultural, and political frameworks and service-delivery mechanisms but also developed a home-grown model, which are local and well-integrated within the Nepali sociostructural environment.

It began with an analysis of the origins of social work in Nepal and its grounding in Indian-influenced US models (see Figures 1.1 and 4.1). Drawing on Nepali social workers' perspectives on this, in the end the book presented a home-grown model of decolonised and developmental Nepali social work that points to the need to shift away from the clinical US and charity-based model towards needs-, welfare-, and rights-based approaches in which community-oriented social work might have an impact on transforming Nepali society, so that all its people can engage in solidary progress to achieve a better quality of life. Rather than self-appointed representatives, the paradigm shift via this model in Nepali social work advocates that democratically elected leaders of social work education would be better equipped to engage relevant government and non-government bodies in a dialogue about the role social work might play in contemporary Nepali society. Further, the model acknowledges that ethnic and indigenous perspectives, as well as culturally relevant practice models, are needed to reach Nepal's diverse cultural and ethnic groups. Such negotiations at the institutional and grassroots levels are needed to achieve the social legitimacy of the social work profession in Nepal.

It takes into consideration a historical perspective that is essential considering past trauma suffered by Nepali peoples and to enhance social workers' understanding of how informal and community-based helping systems have developed to deal with local problems. Likewise, it also makes sense of Nepali peoples' strong connection to environment and spirituality and how they have developed their unique livelihood strategies, kinship and communal solidarity, and ability to cope with adversities. The model has emerged from the Nepali social workers' belief that mutual living and learning from common mistakes go hand and hand where social work mediates between the realities of the past and present to develop the capacities of peoples in the future considering established social norms, values, and practices.

It also explores that Nepali society focuses on blood bonds, responsibilities to the collective family system, and pursuit of grassroots solutions. Also, the country is in a transitional phase following the decade-long Maoist insurgency and is defining human rights, social justice and inclusion, citizens' right to participate in the development agenda, and its democratic process through the newly promulgated constitution. Given these conditions, the model positions that applying a colonial model of social work not only is alienating people from their right to self-determination but also is unethical by Nepali social workers' concerns surrounding cultural relevance.

The form of local, contextual knowledge undergirding the model presented in Chapter 7 reflects Nepali social workers' world views grounded in observation, self-reflection, general knowledge, and lived experience. It gives social work training contextual meaning and direction, and equips social work students with culturally sensitive practice knowledge and tools. It orients social workers to individualise the person in context, culture, and place. It provides an understanding of the multilayered and diverse nature of Nepali society and the social and ethnic divisions that engender conflict and injustice for marginalised groups. It encourages social workers to integrate and partner with other related disciplines to understand the causes and interventions of social issues from a multidisciplinary point of view. It is reflexive and responsive and equips social workers with communication skills to respond flexibly and establish rapport and trust with the populations they serve. It suggests a focus on community development and the importance of establishing strong strategic local connections with community leaders and participatory strategies of community engagement, responsive to local needs and issues.

It suggests that Nepali social work must be multisectoral, dynamic, and community oriented, since collectivism is valued over individualism. Equipping social work with community building and locality development skills to mobilise community members to decide on their own goals and strategies guarantees their autonomy over issues affecting them. Taking into consideration that Nepal is an economically poor country, the model emphasises that Nepal needs a massive production of social workers equipped to deal with poverty within a cultural frame of reference befitting local communities and cultures. It requires culturally relevant practice models to address the needs of Nepal's diverse cultures. Only through a legitimate institutional approach can social work educators and practitioners hope to gain the support of local communities and address poverty at the grassroots level. The terminologies used in both social work and development realms are borrowed and alien to Nepali people. Thus, it is also imperative to develop language of both social work and development sensitive to peoples' day-to-day communication and interactions.

To sum up, it advocates a need for a paradigm shift from Western informed 'Nepalese' to decolonised and developmental 'Nepali' social work that is consistent with the larger social constructionist view in which more than applying my own privileged status as an author, I have valued Nepali social workers' insiders position constructed within Nepali social and structural situations.

Yet, a temporal end

A central purpose of this book, which was to construct a decolonised and developmental Nepali model of social work practice grounded in Nepali social workers' first-hand experiences of working in INGOs and their critical understandings of social work education and practice in Nepal, is just a temporal end. A temporal end in the sense that the model propounded here is not the one finished job, rather just a beginning that must be translated into praxis. And, thus it is relevant to ask: What is the next step in the model of decolonised and developmental Nepali social work? I answer this borrowing from Diversi and Moreira (2009) that

> [the] goal is to arrive in the New Battlegrounds: The decolonizing classroom – the territory for struggle moves from memory to the classroom in the making of new memories of resistance, transformation, notion of inclusiveness. The public performance state – moving from decolonizing discourse toward decolonizing praxis, toward the dream where people come to the academy to do the talking, not the answering: the invasion of the institutional space by the oppressed and marked body, not as object of . . . [Western social work] but as expert of their own struggle.
> (p. 208)

Also, relevant is to ask: How can this be achieved? The decolonised and developmental social work practice requires a curriculum that enables a critical understanding of local problems and issues, and the institutional structures that maintain inequalities and injustices. This includes a deep understanding of cultural diversity and training in culturally responsive social work practice. The curriculum needs to focus on intersectionalities, where social, cultural, economic, and political structures and practices lead to compounded injustices, for example, for women from lower caste groups. To understand how various systems compound disadvantage and maintain social inequities requires a holistic systemic understanding. It is hoped that this book will be applied to the development of the social work curriculum in Nepal and elsewhere that has a similar context.

Worth noting to this end, while this book has drawn on theoretical world views about decolonised and developmental social work practice, there is also a need to develop tangible practice tools and techniques. There is also need to decolonise foreign development discourse from a social work perspective. This book has suggested the need for a socially responsive development paradigm with community development its key method. In the future, social workers need to build partnerships with multiple stakeholders engaged in development to influence local development strategies.

In this book, I have sought to develop a comprehensive model of decolonised and developmental Nepali social work to illustrate that it is possible to synthesise two emerging fields of practice, that is, decolonisation and development. It also argued that 'Nepalisation', that is, first, separation from the Western worldview and, second, Nepali embedded social work, is what required in the Nepali context to respond to contemporary social issues. In ending the book, I have mixed feelings of despair and delight. I feel despair in the sense that I wish to return to the past and craft this book in a completely different manner given the vast intellectual experiences I gathered throughout this scholarly journey. Nevertheless, I also understand at this point that decolonising is an option not a mission (Mignolo & Walsh, 2018); meaning every time I will return to this subject matter I will have new narratives, new discussions, and new analysis to present in new ways. Meanwhile, I feel delight in the sense that a beginning has been marked off to decolonise social work in Nepal, which will transcend the scope and recognition for social work in the country. The Sanskrit quote *anabhyase visham vidya* that I came across at my high school means 'a knowledge without its praxis is like a poison'. This summarises the intention of this scholarly work. Since the time of conception, the broader aim was to reach beyond theoretical knowledge that is applicable in the day-to-day lives of Nepali social workers particularly and others generally. Therefore,

I present this book to you for critique, comment, alteration, adaption, and transfer of the knowledge presented herein. This book showed that a prominent feature of Nepali society was its dynamic normative nature. It is a society that is changing continuously. Future researchers should pay careful attention to time itself, while exploring and situating decolonised and developmental Nepali social work in the future. New dimensions, world views, and methods are, and must be, welcomed as they unfold in the 'new time'. Equally important is to acknowledge the knowledge produced in this book is part of an ongoing process rather than an end, at least this is what my awareness claims:

The beats of decolonisation[1]

Is 'peaceful' instead of 'ultra-radical',
Is 'empirically grounded' instead of 'rational',
Is 'co-construction' instead of 'objectification' of 'participant',
Is 'internally initiated' instead of 'externally imposed',
And, also,
Is 'context bound' instead of 'outside emphasised',
Is 'cultural connection' instead of 'cultural diffusing',
Is 'enduring' instead of 'ending',
Is 'ethical' instead of 'vile',
And above all, is 'solidary' instead of 'competing',

I know, too many things,
Too many ways,
Too many thoughts,
There, in decolonisation,
They are deep,
Deeper in future to build,
That I must keep.

Note

1 Adapted from my own research journal written on February 19, 2015 and modified on August 24, 2018.

References

Adams, J. (1902). *Democracy and social ethics*. New York, NY: Palgrave Macmillan.

Adams, J. (1910). *Twenty Years at Hull House*. New York, NY: Palgrave Macmillan.

Ake, C. (1994). *Democratization of disempowerment in Africa*. Lagos, Nigeria: Malthouse Press.

Al-Dabbagh, A. (1993). Islamic perspectives on social work practice. *American Journal of Islamic Social Science, 10*(4), 536–537.

Al-I Ahmad, J. (2004). Diagnosing an illness. In P. Duara (Ed.), *Decolonization: Perspectives from now and then* (pp. 56–63). New York, NY: Routledge.

Al-Krenawi, A., & Graham, J. R. (1996). Social work and traditional healing rituals among the Bedouin of the Negev, Israel. *International Social Work, 39*(2), 177–188. doi:10.1177/002087289603900206

Al-Krenawi, A., & Graham, J. R. (2001). The cultural mediator: Bridging the gap between a non-western community and professional social work practice. *British Journal of Social Work, 31*(5), 665–685. doi:10.1093/bjsw/31.5.665

Al-Krenawi, A., & Graham, J. R. (2008). Localizing social work with Bedouin-Arab communities in Israel: Limitations and possibilities. In M. Gray, J. Coates, & M. Yellow Bird (Eds.), *Indigenous social work around the world: Towards culturally relevant education and practice*. Aldershot, Hants: Ashgate.

Allan, J., Briskman, L., & Pease, B. (Eds.). (2009). *Critical social work: Theories and practices for a socially just world* (2nd ed.). Crows Nest, NSW: Allen and Unwin.

Alphonse, M., George, P., & Moffatt, K. (2008). Redefining social work standards in the context of globalization: Lessons from India. *International Social Work, 51*, 145–158.

Amnesty International. (2015). *The state of the world's human rights*. London: Amnesty International.

Anfara, V. A., Jr., & Mertz, N. T. (2006). Introduction. In V. A. Anfara, Jr. & N. T. Mertz (Eds.), *Theoretical frameworks in qualitative research* (pp. xii–xxxii). Thousand Oaks, CA: Sage Publications.

The Asia Foundation. (2012). *Political economy analysis of local governance in Nepal with special reference to education health sector*. Kathmandu, Nepal: The Asia Foundation. Retrieved January 26, 2014, from https://asiafoundation.org/resources/pdfs/analysislocalgovernance nepal.pdf

Association of International NGOs. (2014). *AIN membership report 2014*. Kathmandu, Nepal: AIN.

Atal, Y. (1981). The call for indigenization. *International Social Science Journal, 33*(1), 189–197.

Bailey, R. V., & Brake, M. (Eds.). (1975). *Radical social work*. London: Edward Arnold.

Baines, D. (Ed.). (2011). *Doing anti-oppressive practice: Social justice social work* (2nd ed.). Halifax, NS: Fernwood Publishing.

Barise, A. (2005). Social work with Muslims: Insights from the teaching of Islam. *Critical Social Work, 6*(2), 73–89.

Bar-On, A. (2003). Indigenous practice: Some informed guesses-self-evident but impossible. *Social Work-Stellenbosch, 39*(1), 26–40.

Bartlett, R., Bharati, L., Pant, D., Hosterman, H., & McCornick, P. (2010). *Climate change impacts and adaptation in Nepal.* Colombo, Sri Lanka: International Water Management Institute.

Baumgold, D. (1988). *Hobbes's political theory.* New York, NY: Cambridge University Press.

Bell, T. (2014). *Kathmandu.* New Delhi, India: Random House India.

Bennett, L., Dilli, R. D., & Govindasamy, P. (2008). *Caste, ethnic and regional identity in Nepal: Further analysis of the 2006 Nepal demographic and health survey.* Retrieved February 16, 2016, from http://un.org.np/data-coll/Health-Publications/2006_NDHS_Caste_Ethinicity_Identity.pdf

Berger, P. L., & Luckmann, T. (1966). *The social construction of reality: A treatise in the sociology of knowledge.* New York, NY: Anchor.

Berking, H. (1996). Solidary individualism. In S. Lash, B. Szerszynski, & B. Wayne (Eds.), *Risk, environment and modernity.* London: Sage Publications.

Bernstein, B. (1996). *Pedagogy, symbolic control and identity: Theory, research, critique.* London: Taylor & Francis.

Bhandari, S. (2014). *Self-determination and constitution making in Nepal: Constituent Assembly, inclusion, & ethnic federalism.* Singapore: Springer.

Bhattachan, K. B. (1999). NGOs and INGOs in Nepal: Reality and myth. In F. Hossain, M. Ulvila, & W. Newaz (Eds.), *Learning NGOs and the dynamics of development partnership* (pp. 269–280). Dhaka, Bangladesh: Dhaka Ahsania Mission.

Bhattachan, K. B. (2000). Voluntary actions and ethnicity in Nepal: Challenges and limitations. In F. Hossain, J. Vartola, M. Ulvila, & T. N. Dhakal (Eds.), *Development NGOs facing the 21st century perspectives from South Asia* (pp. 74–80). Kathmandu, Nepal: Institute for Human Development.

Bhurtel, J., & Ali, S. H. (n.d.). *The green roots of red rebellion: Environmental degradation and the rise of the Maoist movement in Nepal.* Retrieved July 6, 2014, from www.uvm.edu/~shali/Maoist.pdf?origin=publication_detail

Bhusal, G., & Shahi, Y. (Eds.). (2013). *The left debate in Nepal.* Kathmandu, Nepal: Centre for Nepal Studies and Rosaluxemburg Foundation.

Birks, M., & Mills, J. (2011). *Grounded theory: A practical guide.* Los Angeles, CA: Sage Publications.

Bista, D. B. (1991). *Fatalism and development: Nepal's struggle for modernization.* Calcutta, India: Orient Longman.

Bloodgood, E. A., & Schmitz, H. P. (2013). The INGO research agenda: A community approach to challenges in methods and theory. In B. Reinalda (Ed.), *Routledge handbook of international organizations* (pp. 67–69). New York, NY: Routledge.

Boli, J., & Thomas, G. M. (1999a). INGOs and the organization of world culture. In J. Boli & G. M. Thomas (Eds.), *Constructing world culture: International nongovernmental organizations since 1875* (pp. 13–49). Stanford, CA: Stanford University Press.

Boli, J., & Thomas, G. M. (Eds.). (1999b). *Constructing world culture: International nongovernmental organizations since 1875.* Stanford, CA: Stanford University Press.

Bongartz, H., & Dahal, D. R. (1996). *Development studies: Self-help organizations, NGOs and civil society.* Kathmandu, Nepal: Nepal Foundation for Advanced Studies.

Bonio, F., & Donini, A. (2009). *Aid and violence: Development policies and conflict in Nepal*. Boston, MA: Tufts University.

Boroujerdi, M. (2002). Subduing globalization: The challenge of the indigenization movement. In R. Grant & J. R. Short (Eds.), *Globalization and the margins* (pp. 39–49). New York, NY: Palgrave Macmillan.

Bricker-Jenkins, M., Hooyman, N., & Gottlieb, N. (Eds.). (1991). *Feminist social work practice in clinical settings*. Newbury Park, CA: Sage Publications.

Brieland, D. (1990). The Hull-House tradition and the contemporary social worker: Was Jane Addams really a social worker? *Social Work, 35*(2), 134.

Brinton, C. (1965). *The anatomy of revolution*. New York, NY: Vintage Books.

Briskman, L. (2008). Decolonizing social work in Australia: Prospect or illusion. In M. Gray, J. Coates, & M. Yellow Bird (Eds.), *Indigenous social work around the world: Towards culturally relevant education and practice* (pp. 83–93). Aldershot, Hants: Ashgate.

Brown, M. E. (2001). The causes of internal conflict. In M. E. Brown, O. R. Cote, S. Lynn-Jones, & S. E. Miller (Eds.), *Nationalism and ethnic conflict: An international security reader* (revised ed., pp. 3–25). Cambridge, MA: MIT Press.

Brusset, E., & Regmi, R. R. (2002). *Conflict and development in Nepal*. Kathmandu, Nepal: Department for International Development.

Bruyere, G. (1999). The decolonisation wheel: An aboriginal perspective on social work practice with aboriginal peoples. In R. Delaney, K. Brownlee, & K. Zapf (Eds.), *Social work practice with rural and northern peoples* (pp. 170–181). Thunder Bay, ON: Centre for Northern University Press.

Butler, J. (2002). What is critique? An essay on Foucault's virtue. In D. Ingram (Ed.), *The political: Readings in continental philosophy* (pp. 212–227). Cambridge, MA: Blackwell Publishers.

Butterfield, A. K., & Tasse, A. (Eds.). (2013). *Social development and social work: Learning from Africa*. New York, NY: Routledge.

Canda, E. R. (1988). Conceptualising sprituality for social work: Insights from diverse perspectives. *Social Thoughts, 14*(1), 30–46.

Canda, E. R., & Furman, L. D. (Eds.). (1999). *Spiritual diversity in social work practice: The heart of helping*. New York, NY: Free Press.

Cannella, G. S., & Lincoln, Y. S. (2011). Ethics, research regulations, and critical social science. In N. K. Denzin & Y. S. Lincoln (Eds.), *The Sage handbook of qualitative research* (pp. 81–89). Thousand Oaks, CA: Sage Publications.

Carapico, S. (2000). *NGOs, INGOs, GO-NGOs and DO-NGOs: Making sense of non-governmental organizations: Middle East report*. Richmond, VA: University of Richmond.

Carniol, B. (2005). *Case critical: Social service and social justice in Canada*. Toronto, ON: Between the Lines.

Castells, M. (2000). *End of millennium: The information age: Economy, society and culture* (2nd ed., Vol. 3). Malden, MA: Blackwell Publishers.

Cedric, J. (2009). Democracy. In P. A. Haslam, J. Schafer, & P. Beaudet (Eds.), *Introduction to international development: Approaches, actors, and issues* (pp. 295–312). Oxford, UK: Oxford University Press.

Centre for Economic Development and Administration. (2007). *Financing higher education in Nepal: Final report*. Kathmandu, Nepal: Tribhuvan University.

Chalise, P. (1992). *Nepalko purano itihas ra savyata* [Nepal's old history and civilization]. Kathmandu, Nepal: Ratna Pustak Bhandar.

Chan, K. L., & Chan, C. L. W. (2005). Chinese culture, social work education and research. *International Social Work, 48*(4), 381–389.

Chand, D. (1991). *Development through non-governmental organizations in Nepal*. Kathmandu, Nepal: National Development Research and Social Services.

Chand, D. (2002). *NGO strategy and development of a comprehensive database of development focused NGOs*. Kathmandu, Nepal: Asian Development Bank.

Chang, C. F., & Mo, L. L. (2007). Social work education in Taiwan: Toward professionalism. *Social Work Education, 26*(6), 583–594. doi:10.1080/02615470701456319

Chang, M. (2005). The movement to indigenize the social science in Taiwan: Origin and predicaments. In J. Makeham & A. C. Hsiau (Eds.), *Cultural, ethic, and political nationalism in contemporary Taiwan: Bentuhua* (pp. 221–260). New York, NY: Palgrave Macmillan.

Charmaz, K. (1995a). Between positivism and postmodernism: Implications for methods. In N. K. Denzin (Ed.), *Studies in symbolic interaction* (pp. 43–72). Greenwich, CT: JAI Press.

Charmaz, K. (1995b). Grounded theory. In J. Smith, R. Harre, & L. Langenhove (Eds.), *Rethinking methods in psychology* (pp. 27–65). Thousand Oaks, CA: Sage Publications.

Charmaz, K. (2000). Grounded theory: Objectivist and constructivist methods. In N. Denzin & Y. Lincoln (Eds.), *Handbook of qualitative research* (2nd ed., pp. 509–534). Thousand Oaks, CA: Sage Publications.

Charmaz, K. (2006). *Constructing grounded theory: A practical guide through qualitative analysis*. Thousand Oaks, CA: Sage Publications.

Charmaz, K. (2009). Shifting the grounds: Constructivist grounded theory methods for the twenty-first century. In J. M. Morse, P. N. Stern, J. Corbin, B. Bowers, K. Charmaz, & A. E. Clark (Eds.), *Developing grounded theory: The second generation* (pp. 127–154). Walnut Creek, CA: Left Coast Press.

Charmaz, K. (2011). Grounded theory methods in social justice research. In N. K. Denzin & Y. S. Lincoln (Eds.), *The Sage handbook of qualitative research* (pp. 359–380). Thousand Oaks, CA: Sage Publications.

Charmaz, K., & Mitchell, R. (1996). The myth of silent authorship: Self, substance, and style in ethnogrphic writing. *Symbolic Interaction, 19*(4), 285–302.

Chaturvedy, R. R., & Malone, D. M. (2012). A yam between two boulders: Nepal's foreign policies caught between India and China. In S. von Einsiedel, D. M. Malone, & S. Pradhan (Eds.), *Nepal in transition: From people's war to fragile peace* (pp. 287–312). New Delhi, India: Cambridge University Press.

Cheung, M., & Liu, M. (2004). The self-concept of Chinese women and the indigenization of social work in China. *International Social Work, 47*(1), 109–127. doi:10.1177/002087 2804039390

Clarke, G. (1998). Non-governmental organizations (NGOs) and politics in the developing world. *Political Studies, 46*(1), 36–52. doi:10.1111/1467-9248.00128

Coates, J., Gray, M., & Hetherington, T. (2006). An "ecospiritual" perspective: Finally, a place for indigenous approaches. *British Journal of Social Work, 36*(3), 381–399. doi:10.1093/bjsw/bcl005

Cochran, M. (2010). Dewey as an international thinker. In M. Cochran (Ed.), *The Cambridge companion to Dewey* (pp. 309–338). Cambridge, MA: Cambridge University Press.

Collier, M. J. (2013). Dancing with development: UN and INGO community engagement in Nepal. In M. J. Collier (Ed.), *Community engagement and intercultural praxis: Dancing with difference in diverse contexts* (pp. 31–61). Berne, Switzerland: Peter Lang.

Collier, P., Elliott, V. L., Hegre, H., Reynal-Querol, M., & Sambanis, N. (2003). *Breaking the conflict trap: Civil war and development policy*. Washington, DC: World Bank and Oxford University Press.

Communist Party of Nepal, Maoist. (1995). *Theoretical premises for the historic initiation of the people's war.* Retrieved January 2, 2017, from http://ucpnmaoist.org/PageDetails.aspx?id=340&cat=4-.WGGTSWR96CR

Corrigan, P. (1978). *Social work practice under capitalism: A Marxist approach.* London: Palgrave Macmillan.

Cox, D. (1995). Asia and the pacific. In N. S. Mayadas, T. D. Watts, & D. Elliott (Eds.), *International handbook on social work education* (pp. 321–338). Westport, CT: Greenwood Press.

Crane, S. D. (2002). *The Maoist insurgency in Nepal: 1996–2001.* Carlisle Barracks, PA: U. S. Army War College.

Creswell, J. W. (2009). *Research design: Qualitative, quantitative, and mixed methods approach.* New Delhi, India: Sage Publications.

Crotty, M. (1998). *The foundations of social research: Meaning and perspective in the research process.* Thousand Oaks, CA: Sage Publications.

Dahal, P. (1992). *Nepalko itihas: Suru dekhi Sugali Sandhi Samma* [The history of Nepal: From beginning to the Treaty of Sugauli] (4th ed.). Kathmandu, Nepal: MK Publisher and Distributer.

Dahal, T. N. (2002). *The role of non-governmental organizations in the improvement of livelihood in Nepal* (PhD). Tampere, Finland: University of Tampere.

Dei, G. J. S. (2005). Critical issues in anti-racist research methodology: An introduction. In G. J. S. Dei & G. S. Johal (Eds.), *Critical issues in anti-racist research methodologies* (pp. 1–28). New York, NY: Peter Lang.

Dei, G. J. S., & Johal, G. S. (Eds.). (2005). *Critical issues in anti-racist research methodologies.* New York, NY: Peter Lang.

DeMars, W. (2005). *NGOs and transnational networks: Wild cards in world politics.* London: Pluto Press.

de Urrutia Barroso, L., & Strug, D. (2013). Community-based social work in Cuba. In M. Gray, J. Coates, M. Yellow Bird, & T. Hetherington (Eds.), *Decolonizing social work* (pp. 107–129). Aldershot, Hants: Ashgate.

Devkota, K. (2012). *Dynamics of urbanization in Nepal: The role and response of local government.* Kathmandu, Nepal: Alliance for Social Dialogue.

Devkota, P. L. (2007). Anthropology, society and development in Nepal: A native perspective. *Occasional Papers in Sociology and Anthropology, 7,* 26–40.

Dhakal, T. N. (2006). *NGOs in livelihood improvement Nepalese experience.* New Delhi, India: Adroit Publishers.

Dhakal, T. N. (2007). Challenges of civil society governance in Nepal. *JOAAG, 2*(1), 61–73.

Diamond, L. (1997). In search of consolidation. In L. Diamond, M. F. Plattner, Y. Chu, & H. Tien (Eds.), *Consolidating the third wave democracies: Themes and perspectives* (pp. xiii–xlv). Baltimore, MD: The Johns Hopkins University Press.

Diversi, M., & Moreira, C. (2009). *Betweener talk: Decolonizing knowledge production, pedagogy, and praxis.* Walnut Creek, CA: Left Coast Press.

Dixit, K. (1997). Foreign aid in Nepal: No bang for the buck. *SINHAS, 2*(1), 173–186.

Dominelli, L. (1997). *Anti-racist social work* (2nd ed.). London: Palgrave Macmillan.

Dominelli, L. (1998). Anti-oppresive practice in context. In R. Adams, L. Dominelli, & M. Payne (Eds.), *Social work themes, issues and critical debate* (pp. 3–19). London: Palgrave Macmillan.

Douglas, M. (1996). *Purity and danger.* New York, NY: Routledge.

Downs, H. R. (1980). *Rhythms of a Himalayan village*. New Delhi, India: Book Faith India.

Drucker, D. (1993). The social work profession in Asia: A look homeward 1968–1993. *The Indian Journal of Social Work*, *54*(4), 513–536.

DuBois, W. E. B. (1961). *The souls of black folks: Essays and sketches*. New York, NY: Fawcett Publications.

Duffield, M. (2014). *Global governance and the new wars: The merging of development and security*. New York, NY: Zed Books.

Durkheim, E. (1997). *The division of labor in society* (W. D. Halls, Trans.). New York, NY: The Free Press.

Elliott, D. (1993). Social work and social development: Towards an integrative model of social work practice. *International Social Work*, *36*(1), 21–36.

Engel, R. J., & Schutt, R. K. (2013). *The practice of research in social work* (3rd ed.). Thousand Oaks, CA: Sage Publications.

Esteva, G. (1992). Development. In W. Sachs (Ed.), *The development dictionary: A guide to knowledge as power* (pp. 6–26). New York, NY: Zed Books.

Evetts, J. (1998). Professionalism beyond the nation-state: International systems of professional regulation in Europe. *International Journal of Sociology and Policy*, *18*(11/12), 47–64.

Fanon, F. (1986). *Black skin white masks* (C. L. Markmann, Trans.). London: Pluto Press.

Ferguson, H. (2002). Social work, individualization and life politics. *British Journal of Social Work*, *31*(1), 45–55.

Ferguson, K. M. (2005). Beyond indigenization and reconceptualization: Towards a global, multidirectional model of technology transfer. *International Social Work*, *48*(5), 519–535.

Finnemore, M., & Sikkink, K. (1998). International norm dynamics and political change. *International Organization*, *52*(4), 887–917.

Fisher, W. F. (1997). Doing good? The politics and anti-politics of NGO practices. *Annual Review of Anthropology*, *26*, 439–464.

Food and Agriculture Organization of the United Nations. (2010). *Global forest resources assessment 2010*. Rome: FAO.

Foucault, M. (1984). What is enlightenment? (C. Porter, Trans.). In P. Rainbow (Ed.), *The Foucault reader* (pp. 32–50). New York, NY: Vintage Books.

Franklin, J. H. (1978). *John Locke and the theory of sovereignty: Mixed monarchy and the right of resistance in the political thought of the English revolution*. New York, NY: Cambridge University Press.

Freedom House. (2015). *Freedom in the world 2015*. Washington, DC: Freedom House.

Freire, P. (1974). *Pedagogy of the oppressed*. New York, NY: Continuum.

Fujikura, T. (2001). Discourse of awareness: Notes for a criticism of development in Nepal. *Studies in Nepali History & Society*, *6*(2), 271–313.

Gandhi, L. (1998). *Postcolonial theory: A critical introduction*. New York, NY: Columbia University Press.

Gaztambide-Fernández, R. A. (2012). Decolonization and the pedagogy of solidarity. *Decolonization: Indigeneity, Education & Society*, *1*(1), 41–67.

Gellner, D. N. (2007). *Democracy in Nepal: Four models*. Seminar 576. Retrieved September 23, 2013, from www.uni-bielefeld.de/midea/pdf/darticle3.pdf

Gellner, D. N. (2010). Caste, ethnicity and inequality in Nepal. *Economic and Political Weekly*, *42*(20), 1823–1828.

Gellner, D. N., & Hachhethu, K. (Eds.). (2008). *Local democracy in South Asia: Microprocesses of democratization in Nepal and its neighbours*. London: Sage Publications.

Ghimire, Y. (2015). Protests against India in Nepal: The big brother syndrome? *The Indian Express*. Retrieved October 8, 2016, from http://indianexpress.com/article/explained/protests-against-india-in-nepal-the-big-brother-syndrome/

Gilgun, J. F. (2011). Grounded theory and other inductive research methods. In B. A. Thyer (Ed.), *The handbook of social work research methods* (pp. 345–364). London: Sage Publications.

Gilgun, J. F., & Abrams, L. S. (2002). The nature and usefulness of qualitative social work research: Some thoughts and an invitation to dialogue. *Qualitative Social Work*, *1*(1), 39–55. doi:10.1177/1473325002001001743

Gilligun, P., & Furness, S. (2005). The role of religion and spirituality in social work practice: Views and experiences of social workers and students. *British Journal of Social Work*, *36*(4), 617–637.

Giulianotti, R., & Robertson, R. (2009). *Globalization and football*. London: Sage Publications.

Glaser, B. G. (1978). *Theoretical sensitivity: Advances in the methodology of grounded theory*. Mill Valley, CA: Sociology Press.

Glaser, B. G., & Strauss, A. (1967). *The discovery of grounded theory*. Chicago, IL: Aldine.

Glesne, C. (2007). Research as solidarity. In N. K. Denzin & M. D. Giardina (Eds.), *Ethical futures in qualitative research: Decolonizing the politics of knowledge* (pp. 169–178). Walnut Creek, CA: Left Coast Press.

Gordon, S. (1991). *The history and philosophy of social science*. New York, NY: Routledge.

Gould, H. A. (1961). Sanskritization and westernization: A dynamic view. *Economic Weekly*, *13*(25), 945–950.

Government of Nepal. (1956). *The first five-year plan 1956–1961*. Kathmandu, Nepal: GoN.

Government of Nepal. (1961). *National Directive Act 1962* § 3 (1962).

Government of Nepal. (1962a). *Foreign Exchange (Regulation) Act 1962* § 3.

Government of Nepal. (1962b). *The second three-year plan 1962–1965*. Kathmandu, Nepal: GoN.

Government of Nepal. (1965). *The third five-year plan 1965–1970*. Kathmandu, Nepal: GoN.

Government of Nepal. (1970). *The fourth five-year plan 1970–1975*. Kathmandu, Nepal: GoN.

Government of Nepal. (1971). *The national education system plan for 1971–76*. Kathmandu, Nepal: Ministry of Education.

Government of Nepal. (1975). *The fifth five-year plan 1975–1980*. Kathmandu, Nepal: GoN.

Government of Nepal. (1977). *Society Registration Act 1977* §§ 2–12.

Government of Nepal. (1980). *The sixth five-year plan 1980–1985*. Kathmandu, Nepal: GoN.

Government of Nepal. (1985). *The seventh five-year plan 1985–1990*. Kathmandu, Nepal: GoN.

Government of Nepal. (1991). *The eighth plan 1991–1996*. Kathmandu, Nepal: GoN.

Government of Nepal. (1992a). *The Social Welfare Act, 2049*.

Government of Nepal. (1992b). *The Village Development Committee Act, 2049* § 26.

Government of Nepal. (1997). *The ninth five-year plan 1997–2002*. Kathmandu, Nepal: GoN.

Government of Nepal. (1999). *Local Self-Governance Act 1999* §§ 28–163. Kathmandu, Nepal: GoN.

Government of Nepal. (2003). *The tenth plan (poverty reeducation strategy paper) 2000–2007*. Kathmandu, Nepal: NPC.

Government of Nepal. (2008). *The interim three year plan (2007/8–2009/10).* Kathmandu, Nepal: NPC.

Government of Nepal. (2011a). *Nepal living standards survey 2010/11, statistical report* (Vol. 1). Kathmandu, Nepal: NPC.

Government of Nepal. (2011b). *Nepal population report 2011.* Kathmandu, Nepal: Ministry of Health and Population.

Government of Nepal. (2011c). *Twelfth plan 2010/11–2012/13.* Kathmandu, Nepal: NPC.

Government of Nepal. (2012a). *Assessment of social security allowance program in Nepal.* Kathmandu, Nepal: NPC. Retrieved May 13, 2014, from www.npc.gov.np/new/uploaded Files/allFiles/SSAP_Detail_Book.pdf

Government of Nepal. (2012b). *National population and housing census.* Kathmandu, Nepal: GoN.

Government of Nepal. (2014). *Thirteenth plan 2013/14–2015/16.* Kathmandu, Nepal: NPC.

Government of Nepal. (2015). *Constitution of Nepal.* Kathmandu, Nepal: GoN.

Government of Nepal. (2017). *Provinces of Nepal.* Kathmandu, Nepal: Electoral Constituency Delineation Commission. Retrieved July 23, 2018, from www.election.gov.np/ecn/uploads/userfiles/maps/NEPAL_PROVINCEMAP.pdf

Government of Nepal, & United Nations Development Program. (2014). *Nepal human development report 2014: Beyond geography, unlocking human potential.* Kathmandu, Nepal: NPC and UNDP.

Government of Nepal, & United Nations Nepal. (2013). *Nepal millennium development goals: Progress report 2013.* Kathmandu, Nepal: NPC and United Nations Country Team Nepal.

Graham, J. R., Al-Krenawi, A., & Zaidi, S. (2007). Social work in Pakistan: Preliminary insights. *International Social Work, 50*(5), 627–640. doi:10.1177/002087280 7079920

Grande, S. (2007). Red pedagogy: Indigenizing inquiry or the un-methodology. In N. K. Denzin & M. D. Giardina (Eds.), *Ethical futures in qualitative research: Decolonizing the politics of knowledge* (pp. 133–144). Walnut Creek, CA: Left Coast Press.

Gray, M. (2000). Social work and the "social service professions". *Social Work/Maatskaplike Werk, 36*(1), 99–109.

Gray, M. (2002). Developmental social work: A "strength" praxis for social development. *Social Development Issues, 24*(1), 4–14.

Gray, M. (2005). Dilemmas of international social work: Paradoxical processes in indigenisation, universalism and imperialism. *International Journal of Social Welfare, 14*(2), 230–237.

Gray, M., & Coates, J. (2008). From "indigenization" to cultural relevance. In M. Gray, J. Coates, & M. Yellow Bird (Eds.), *Indigenous social work around the world: Towards culturally relevant education and practice* (pp. 13–30). Aldershot, Hants: Ashgate.

Gray, M., & Coates, J. (2010). "Indigenization" and knowledge development: Extending the debate. *International Social, 53*(5), 1–15.

Gray, M., Coates, J., & Yellow Bird, M. (2008a). Introduction. In M. Gray, J. Coates, & M. Yellow Bird (Eds.), *Indigenous social work around the world: Towards culturally relevant education and practice* (pp. 1–12). Aldershot, Hants: Ashgate.

Gray, M., Coates, J., & Yellow Bird, M. (Eds.). (2008b). *Indigenous social work around the world: Towards culturally relevant education and practice.* Aldershot, Hants: Ashgate.

Gray, M., Coates, J., Yellow Bird, M., & Hetherington, T. (2013a). Conclusion: Continuing the decolonization agenda. In M. Gray, J. Coates, M. Yellow Bird, & T. Hetherington (Eds.), *Decolonizing social work* (pp. 323–332). Aldershot, Hants: Ashgate.

Gray, M., Coates, J., Yellow Bird, M., & Hetherington, T. (2013b). Introduction: Scoping the terrain of decolonization. In M. Gray, J. Coates, M. Yellow Bird, & T. Hetherington (Eds.), *Decolonizing social work* (pp. 1–14). Aldershot, Hants: Ashgate.

Gray, M., Coates, J., Yellow Bird, M., & Hetherington, T. (Eds.). (2013c). *Decolonising social work*. Aldershot, Hants: Ashgate.

Gray, M., & Hetherington, T. (2013). Indigenization, indigenous social work and decolonization: Mapping the theoretical terrain. In M. Gray, J. Coates, M. Yellow Bird, & T. Hetherington (Eds.), *Decolonizing social work* (pp. 25–42). Aldershot, Hants: Ashgate.

Gray, M., & Webb, S. A. (2013a). Introduction. In M. Gray & S. A. Webb (Eds.), *Social work theories and methods* (2nd ed., pp. 1–10). London: Sage Publications.

Gray, M., & Webb, S. A. (Eds.). (2013b). *The new politics of social work*. Basingstoke, Hants: Palgrave Macmillan.

Gray, M., & Webb, S. A. (2014). No issue, no politics: Towards a new left in social work education. In C. Noble, H. Strauss, & B. Littlechild (Eds.), *Global social work: Crossing borders, blurring boundaries* (pp. 327–340). Sydney, NSW: Sydney University Press.

Gray, M., & Yadav, R. K. (2015). Social work without borders: A janus-faced concept. *Social Dialogue, 11*, 28–29.

Gray, M., Yellow Bird, M., & Coates, J. (2008). Towards an understanding of indigenous social work. In M. Gray, J. Coates, & M. Yellow Bird (Eds.), *Indigenous social work around the world: Towards culturally relevant education and practice* (pp. 49–58). Aldershot, Hants: Ashgate.

Green, J. W. (1982). *Cultural awareness in the human service*. Englewood Cliffs, NJ: Prentice-Hall.

Green, J. W. (1999). *Cultural awareness in the human service: A multi-ethnic approach* (3rd ed.). Needham Heights, MA: Allyn and Bacon.

Greetz, C. (1983). *Local knowledge: Further essays in interpretive anthropology*. New York, NY: Basic Books.

Gregor, S. (2006). The nature of theory in information system. *MIS Quarterly, 30*(3), 611–641.

Greif, G. L. (2004). How international is the social work knowledge base? *Social Work, 49*(3), 514–516. doi:10.1093/sw/49.3.514

Griffin, P. (2009). *Gendering the World Bank: Neoliberalism and the gendered foundations of global governance*. New York, NY: Palgrave Macmillan.

Guba, E. G., & Lincoln, Y. S. (1985). *Naturalistic inquiry*. Newbury Park, CA: Sage Publications.

Gurung, H. (2002). Trident and thunderbolt: Cultural dynamics in Nepali politics. In B. K. Battachan (Ed.), *Ethnicity, caste and a pluralist society*. Kathmandu, Nepal: Social Science Baha Himal Association.

Gurung, H. (2005). The Dalit context. *Occasional Papers in Sociology Anthropology, 9*, 1–27.

Gurung, H. (2006). *Social inclusion and nation building in Nepal*. Paper presented at the Civil Society Forum Workshop, Lalitpur. Retrieved February 11, 2014, from www.social inclusion.org.np/new/files/Social%20Inclusion%20and%20Nation%20Building%20 in%20Nepal%20-%20Dr%20Hakra%20Gurung_1336541331c25e.pdf

Gurung, O. (2009). Social inclusion: Policies and practices in Nepal. *Occasional Papers in Sociology and Anthropology, 11*, 1–15.

Habermas, J. (1987). *Knowledge and human interests* (J. Shapiro, Trans.). Maiden, MA: Polity Press.

Hachhethu, K. (1997). Nepal in 1996. *Asian Survey, 37*(2), 149–154.

Hafner-Burton, E. M. (2008). Sticks and stones: Naming and shaming the human rights enforcement problem. *International Organization, 62*(4), 689–716. doi:10.1017/S0020818308080247

Haj-Yahia, M. M. (1997). Culturally sensitive supervision of Arab social work students in Western students. *Social Work, 42*, 166–174.

Hamilton, F. B. (1819). *An account of kingdom of Nepal and of the territories annexed to this domain by the house of Gurkha*. Edinburgh, Scotland: Archibald Constable and Company.

Hangen, S. I. (2009). *The rise of ethnic politics in Nepal: Democracy in the margins*. Hoboken, NJ: Taylor & Francis.

Hanlon, J., Barrientos, A., & Hulme, D. (2010). *Just give money to the poor: The development revolution from the Global South*. West Hartford, CT: Kumarian Press.

Hardcastle, D., Wenocur, S., & Powers, P. R. (1997). *Community practice: Theories and skills for social workers*. New York, NY: Oxford University Press.

Harris, B. (2006). A first nations perspective on social justice in social work: Are we there yet? (A post-colonial debate). *The Canadian Journal of Native Studies, 26*(2), 229–263.

Harris, J., & Chou, Y.-C. (2001). Globalization or glocalization? Community care in Taiwan and Britain. *European Journal of Social Work, 4*(2), 161–172.

Hart, M. A. (2009). For indigenous people, by indigenous people, with indigenous people towards an indigenist research paradigm. In R. Sinclair, M. A. Hart, & G. Bruyere (Eds.), *Wicihitowin: Aboriginal social work in Canada* (pp. 153–169). Halifax, NS: Fernwood Publishing.

Haug, E. (2005). Critical reflections on the emerging discourse of international social work. *International Social Work, 48*(2), 126–135.

Healy, L. M., & Link, R. (Eds.). (2012). *Handbook of international social work: Human rights, development, and the global profession*. New York, NY: Oxford University Press.

Hetherington, T. (2009). *Indigenous social work: A comparative study of New Brunswick (Canada) and Alice Springs (Australia)* (Doctoral). Newcastle, Australia: The University of Newcastle.

Hick, S. F. (2009). *Structural social work*. London: Sage Publications.

Hodge, D. R., & Nadir, A. (2008). Moving toward culturally competent practice with Muslims: Modifying cognitive therapy with Islamic tenets. *Social Work, 53*(1), 31–41. doi:10.1093/sw/53.1.31

Hodson, B. H. (1817). *Essays on the language, literature, and religion of Nepal and Tibet*. London: Trubner and Company.

Högger, R. (1997). *Naga and Garuda: The other side of development aid*. Kathmandu, Nepal: Sahayogi Press.

Holtzhausen, L. (2011). When values collide: Finding common ground for social work education in the United Arab Emirates. *International Social Work, 54*(2), 191–208. doi:10.1177/0020872810372364

Hudock, A. C. (1999). *NGOs and civil society: Democracy by proxy*. Cambridge, MA: Polity Press.

Hugman, R. (2016). *Social development in social work: Practices and principles*. New York, NY: Routledge.

Human Rights Treaty Monitoring Coordination Committee. (2008). *Nepal: Status of ratification of key international instruments*. Retrieved April 22, 2014, from www.inseconline.org/files/documents/Nepal_Treaties.pd

Hurdle, D. E. (2002). Native Hawaiian traditional healing: Culturally based interventions for social work practice. *Social Work, 47*(2), 183–192.

Hutt, M. (Ed.). (2004). *Himalayan people's war: Nepal's Maoist rebellion*. Bloomington, IN: Indiana University Press.

Ife, J. (1995). *Community development: Creating community alternatives-vision, analysis and practice*. Melbourne, VIC: Longman.

Ife, J. (2013). *Community development in an uncertain world*. Port Melbourne, VIC: Cambridge University Press.

Ingram, D. (2018). *World crisis and underdevelopment: A critical theory of poverty, agency, and coercion*. New York, NY: Cambridge University Press.

Integrated Regional Information Networks. (2010). *Disadvantaged children missing out on education*. Retrieved March 7, 2014, from www.irinnews.org/fr/ node/248693

International Association for Schools of Social Work, International Council on Social Welfare, & International Federation of Social Workers. (2016). *Global agenda for social work and social development: Second report: Promoting the dignity and worth of peoples*. Berne, Switzerland: IFSW.

International Federation of Social Workers. (2017). *Our members*. Retrieved May 20, 2017, from http://ifsw.org/membership/our-members/

International Fund for Agriculture Development. (2014). *Enabling poor rural people to overcome poverty in Nepal*. Retrieved November 7, 2015, from www.ifad.org/operations/projects/regions/pi/factsheets/nepal.pdf

International Labour Organization. (2013). *The ILO in Nepal*. Retrieved November 26, 2015, from www.ilo.org/wcmsp5/groups/public/-asia/-ro-bangkok/-ilo-kathmandu/documents/publication/wcms_360563.pdf

Ishii, H., & Karan, P. P. (1997). *Nepal: A Himalayan kingdom in transition*. New Delhi, India: Bookwell.

Ives, N. G., & Loft, M. T. (2013). Building bridges with indigenous communities through social work education. In M. Gray, J. Coates, M. Yellow Bird, & T. Hetherington (Eds.), *Decolonizing social work* (pp. 237–255). Aldershot, Hants: Ashgate.

James, A. L. (2004). The McDonaldization of social work: Or "come back florence hollis, all is (or should be) forgiven". In R. Lovelock, K. Lyons, & J. Powell (Eds.), *Reflecting on social work: Discipline and profession* (pp. 37–54). Burlington, VT: Ashgate.

Janesick, V. J. (2000). The choreography of qualitative research design. In N. K. Denzin & Y. S. Lincoln (Eds.), *Handbook of qualitative research* (pp. 379–399). Thousand Oaks, CA: Sage Publications.

Jenlink, E. P. (2004). Education, social creativity and evolution of society. *World Futures*, *60*(3), 225–240.

Jha, P. (2012). A Nepali perspective on international involvement in Nepal. In S. von Einsiedel, D. M. Malone, & S. Pradhan (Eds.), *Nepal in transition: From people's war to fragile peace* (pp. 332–360). New Delhi, India: Cambridge University Press.

Jinchao, Y. (1995). The developing models of social work education in China. *International Social Work*, *38*, 27–38.

Johnston-Goodstar, K. (2013). Indigenous youth participatory action research: Re-visioning social justice for social work with indigenous youths. *Social Work*, *58*(4), 314–320. doi:10.1093/sw/swt036

Jones, L., & Boyd, E. (2011). Exploring social barriers to adaptation: Insights from Western Nepal. *Global Environmental Change*, *21*(4), 1262–1274. doi:10.1016/j.gloenvcha.2011.06.002

Jürgen, O. (1997). *Colonialism: A theoretical overview* (S. L. Frisch, Trans.). Princeton, NJ: Markus Wiener Publishers.

Karan, P. P., & Ishii, H. (1994). *Nepal: Development and change in a landlocked Himalayan kingdom*. Tokyo, Japan: Tokyo University of Foreign Studies.

Keck, M. E., & Sikkink, K. (1998). *Activists beyond borders: Advocacy networks in international politics*. London: Cornell University Press.

Kenny, S. (2010). *Developing communities for the future* (4th ed.). South Melbourne, VIC: Thomson.

Kernot, S. (2006). Nepal: A development challenge. *South Asia: Journal of South Asian Studies*, *29*(2), 293–307. doi:10.1080/00856400600849167

Khadka, N. (1991). *Foreign aid, poverty, and stagnation in Nepal*. New Delhi, India: Vikas Pub. House.

Khan, M. H. (2002, June 24–26). *State failure in developing countries and strategies of institutional reform*. Paper presented at the Annual Bank Conference on Development Economies, Oslo, Norway.

Kharel, K. (2013). Overhauling social work education. *Republica*, 13. Retrieved August 4, 2013, from http://e.myrepublica.com/component/flippingbook/book/1199-republica-03-april-2013/1-republica.html

Khinduka, S. K. (1971). Social work and the Third World. *Social Service Review, 45*(1), 62–73. doi:10.2307/30021784

Khinduka, S. K. (2007). Toward rigor and relevance in US social work education. *Australian Social Work, 60*(1), 18–28.

Kimuyu, P. (1999). *Development policy in Kenya: Which way forward?* Retrieved March 23, 2014, from http://web.peacelink.it/wajibu/7_issue/p1.html

Kincheloe, J. L. (2007). Critical pedagogy in the twenty-first century. In P. McLaren & J. L. Kincheloe (Eds.), *Critical pedagogy: Where are we now?* (pp. 9–42). New York, NY: Peter Lang.

Kirk Patric, C. W. (1811). *An account of the kingdom of Nepal*. London: William Miller.

Korten, D. C. (1990). *Getting to the 21st century: Voluntary action and global agenda*. Hartford, CT: Kumarian Press.

Kovach, M. (2005). Emerging from the Margins: Indigenous methodologies. In L. A. Brown & S. Strega (Eds.), *Research as resistance: Critical, indigenous and anti-oppressive approach*. Toronto, ON: Canadian Scholar's Press.

Kovach, M. (2009). *Indigenous methodologies: Characteristics, conversations and contexts*. Toronto, ON: University of Toronto Press.

Kulkarni, P. D. (1993). The indigenous-base of social work profession in India. *Indian Journal of Social Work, 54*(4), 555–565.

Kumar, D. (2000). What ails democracy in Nepal? In D. Kumar (Ed.), *Domestic conflict and crisis of governability in Nepal* (pp. 14–57). Kathmandu, Nepal: CNAS.

Lake, D. A. (2010). Building legitimate states after civil wars. In M. Hoddie & C. A. Hartzell (Eds.), *Strengthening peace in post-civil war states: Transforming spoilers into stakeholders* (pp. 29–52). Chicago, IL: University of Chicago Press.

Lavalette, M. (Ed.). (2011). *Radical social work today: Social work at the crossroads*. Bristol, UK: Policy Press.

Lawoti, M. (2003). Centralizing politics and the growth of the Maoist insurgency in Nepal. *Himalaya, 13*(1), 49–58.

Lawoti, M. (2005). *Towards a democratic Nepal: Inclusive political institutions for a multicultural society*. London: Sage Publications.

Lawoti, M. (2010). Evolution and growth of the Maoist insurgency in Nepal. In M. Lawoti & A. K. Pahari (Eds.), *The Maoist insurgency in Nepal: Revolution in the twenty-first century* (pp. 3–30). New York, NY: Routledge.

Lawoti, M. (2012). Ethnic politics and the building of an inclusive state. In S. V. Einsiedel, D. M. Malone, & S. Pradhan (Eds.), *Nepal in transition: From people's war to fragile peace* (pp. 129–152). New Delhi, India: Cambridge University Press.

Lawoti, M., & Pahari, A. K. (Eds.). (2010). *The Maoist Insurgency in Nepal: Revolution in the twenty-first century*. New York, NY: Routledge.

Lewis, D., & Kanji, N. (2009). *Non-governmental organizations and development*. New York, NY: Routledge.

Li, Y., Han, W.-J., & Huang, C.-C. (2012). Development of social work education in China: Background, current status, and prospects. *Journal of Social Work Education, 48*(4), 635–653. doi:10.5175/JSWE.2012.201100049

Ling, H. K. (2003). Drawing lessons from local designated helpers to develop culturally appropriate social work practice. *Asia Pacific Journal of Social Work, 13*(2), 26–45.

Ling, H. K. (2004). The search from within: Research issues in relation to developing culturally appropriate social work practice. *International Social Work, 47*(3), 336–345.

Ling, H. K. (2008). The development of culturally appropriate social work practice in Sarawak, Malaysia. In M. Gray, J. Coates, & M. Yellow Bird (Eds.), *Indigenous social work around the world: Towards culturally relevant education and practice* (pp. 97–106). Aldershot, Hants: Ashgate.

Locke, J. (1821). *Two treaties of government.* London: Whitmore and Fenn.

Lofland, J., & Lofland, L. H. (1995). *Analyzing social settings: A guide to qualitative observation and analysis* (3rd ed.). Belmont, CA: Wadsworth Publishing Company.

Loomis, T. M. (2000). Indigenous populations and sustainable development: Building on indigenous approaches to holistic, self-determined development. *World Development, 28*(5), 893–910.

Luger, K., & Höivik, S. (2004). With reverence for culture and nature: Development and modernization in the Himalaya. In A. Loseries-Leick & F. Horvath (Eds.), *Path to nature's wisdom: Ecological dialogue Himalaya & Alps* (pp. 145–166). Graz, Austria: Naturschutzbund Steiermark.

Lum, D. (1999). *Culturally competence practice: A framework for growth and action.* Pacific Grove, CA: Brooks and Cole.

Lundblad, K. S. (1995). Jane Adams and social reform: A role model for the 1990s. *Social Work, 40*(5), 661–669.

Macdonald, L. (1994). Globalizing civil society: Interpreting international NGOs in Central America. *Millennium: Journal of International Studies, 23*(2), 267–285.

Maclure, R., Sabbah, R., & Lavan, D. (2009). Education and development: The perennial contradictions of policy discourse. In P. A. Haslam, J. Schafer, & P. Beaudet (Eds.), *Introduction to international development: Approaches, actors, and issues.* New York, NY: Oxford University Press.

Mafile'o, T. (2008). Tongan social work practice. In M. Gray, J. Coates, & M. Yellow Bird (Eds.), *Indigenous social work around the world: Towards culturally relevant education and practice* (pp. 117–128). Aldershot, Hants: Ashgate.

Mahdavy, H. (1970). The pattern and problems of economic development in rentier states: The case of Iran. In M. A. Cook (Ed.), *Studies in the economic history of the Middle East* (pp. 428–467). Oxford, UK: Oxford University Press.

Mandal, K. S. (1989). American influence on social work education in India and its impact. *Economic and Political Weekly, 24*(49), 2710–2712. doi:10.2307/43956 83

Manuel, G., & Posluns, M. (1974). *The fourth world: An Indian reality.* New York, NY: Free Press.

Marais, L., & Marais, L. C. (2007). Walking between worlds: An exploration of the interface between indigenous and first-world industrialized culture. *International Social Work, 50*(6), 809–820. doi:10.1177/0020872807081920

Martin, I. (2012). The United Nations and support to Nepal's peace process: The role of the UN Mission in Nepal. In S. von Einsiedel, D. M. Malone, & S. Pradhan (Eds.), *Nepal in transition: From people's war to fragile peace* (pp. 201–231). New Delhi, India: Cambridge University Press.

Martinez-Brawley, E. E., & Zorita, P. M.-B. (1998). At the edge of the frame: Beyond science and art in social work. *British Journal of Social Work, 28*(2), 197–212.

Mathou, T. (2005). Tibet and its neighbours: Moving toward a new Chinese strategy in the Himalayan region. *Asian Survey, 45*(4), 517–518.

Matsuoka, J. K., Morelli, P. T., & McCubbin, H. (2013). Indigenizing research for culturally relevant social work practice. In M. Gray, J. Coates, M. Yellow Bird, & T. Hetherington (Eds.), *Decolonizing social work* (pp. 271–292). Aldershot, Hants: Ashgate.

Mayadas, N. S., & Elliott, D. (1997). Lessons from international social work: Policies and practices. In M. Reisch & E. Gambrill (Eds.), *Social work in the 21st century* (pp. 175–185). Thousand Oaks, CA: Pine Forge Press.

McDonald, C., Harris, J., & Wintersteen, R. (2003). Contingent on context? Social work and the state in Australia, Britain and the USA. *British Journal of Social Work, 33*, 191–208.

McLaren, P. (1988). On ideology and education: Critical pedagogy and the politics of education. *Social Text, 19 & 20*, 153–185.

Michels, R. (1915). *Political parties: A Sociological study of the oligarchical tendencies of modern democracy* (E. Paul & C. Paul, Trans.). Kitchener, ON: Batoche Books.

Midgley, J. (1981). *Professional imperialism: Social work in the Third World*. London: Heinemann Educational Books Ltd.

Midgley, J. (2008). Promoting reciprocal international social work exchanges: Professional imperialism revisited. In M. Gray, J. Coates, & M. Yellow Bird (Eds.), *Indigenous social work around the world: Towards culturally relevant education and practice* (pp. 31–45). Aldershot, Hants: Ashgate.

Midgley, J. (2014). *Social development: Theory and practice*. Los Angeles, CA: Sage Publications.

Midgley, J., & Conley, A. (Eds.). (2010). *Social work and social development: Theories and skills for developmental social work*. New York, NY: Oxford University Press.

Migdal, J. S. (1988). *Strong societies and weak states: State-society relations and state capabilities in the Third World*. Princeton, NJ: Princeton University Press.

Mignolo, W. D. (2012). Decolonizing Western epistemology/Building decolonial epistemology. In A. M. Isasi-Diaz & E. Mendieta (Eds.), *Decolonizing epistemologies: Latina/o theology and philosophy* (pp. 19–43). New York, NY: Fordham University.

Mignolo, W. D., & Walsh, C. E. (2018). *On decoloniality: Concepts, analytics, praxis*. London: Duke University Press.

Mills, J., Bonner, A., & Francis, K. (2006). The development of constructivist grounded theory. *International Journal of Qualitative Methods, 5*(1), 1–10.

Mishra, C. (2007). Foreign aid and social structure: Notes on the intrastate relationship. In C. Mishra (Ed.), *Essays on the sociology of Nepal* (pp. 163–174). Kathmandu, Nepal: Fine Print Books.

Mittra, S., & Kumar, B. (2004). *Encyclopaedia of women in South Asia: Nepal* (Vol. 6). New Delhi, India: Kalpaz Publishers.

Mohan, B. (1993). Diversity and conflict: Towards a unified model of social work. *Indian Journal of Social Work, 54*(4), 596–608.

Mokuau, N., & Mataira, P. J. (2013). From trauma to triumph: Perspectives for native Hawaiin and Maori peoples. In M. Gray, J. Coates, M. Yellow Bird, & T. Hetherington (Eds.), *Decolonizing social work* (pp. 145–164). Aldershot, Hants: Ashgate.

Morley, C. (2014). *Engaging with social work: A critical introduction*. Melbourne, VIC: Cambridge University Press.

Mosse, D. (Ed.). (2011). *Adventures in aidland: The anthropology of professionals in international development*. New York, NY: Berghahn Books.

Mozaffar, S. (2010). States and civil societies following civil wars. In M. Hoddie & C. A. Hart (Eds.), *Strengthening peace in post-civil war states: Transforming spoilers into stakeholders* (pp. 53–78). Chicago, IL: University of Chicago Press.

Mukundarao, K. (1969). Social work in India: Indigenous culture base and the process of indigenization. *International Social Work, 12*, 29–39.

Mullaly, B. (2002). *Challenging oppression: A critical social work approach.* Toronto, ON: Oxford University Press.

Mullaly, B. (2009). *Challenging oppression and confronting privilege.* Toronto, ON: Oxford University Press.

Mullaly, R. P. (1997). *Structural social work: Ideology, theory, and practice* (2nd ed.). New York, NY: Oxford University Press.

Munck, R. (1999). Deconstructing development discourses: Of impasses, alternatives and politics. In R. Munck & D. O'Hearn (Eds.), *Critical development theory: Contribution to a new paradigm* (pp. 196–210). New York, NY: Zed Books.

Muni, S. D. (2012). Bringing the Maoist down from the hills: India's role. In S. von Einsiedel, D. M. Malone, & S. Pradhan (Eds.), *Nepal in transition: From people's war to fragile peace* (pp. 313–331). New Delhi, India: Cambridge University Press.

Murdie, A. (2014). *Help or harm: The human security effects of international NGOs.* Stanford, CA: Stanford University Press.

Murdie, A., & Davis, D. R. (2012). Looking in the mirror: Comparing INGO networks across issue areas. *Review of International Organizations, 7*(2), 177–202.

Murshed, S. M., & Gates, S. (2005). Spatial-horizontal inequality and the Maoist insurgency in Nepal. *Review of Development Economics, 9*(1), 121–134. doi:10.1111/j.1467-9361.2005.00267.x

Nagpaul, H. (1972). The diffusion of American social work education to India: Problems and issues. *International Social Work, 15*(1), 3–17. doi:10.1177/002 087287201500103

Nagpaul, H. (1993). Analysis of social work teaching material in India: The need for indigenous foundations. *International Social Work, 36,* 207–220.

Nanavathy, M. C. (1993). Problems affecting the indigenization of social work profession in Asia. *The Indian Journal of Social Work, 54*(5), 547–554.

National Human Rights Commission of Nepal, & Office of the High Commissioner for Human Rights in Nepal. (2011). *Indicators for monitoring economic, social and cultural rights in Nepal: A user's manual.* Kathmandu, Nepal: National Human Rights Commission, Nepal.

Netting, F. E., Kettner, P. M., & McMurtry, S. L. (2004). *Social work macro practice.* Boston, MA: Pearson.

Neupane, G. (2005). *Nepalko jatiya prashna: Samajik banot ra sajhedariko sambandha ma* [Question on Nepali caste system: Relating social structure and collaboration] (Revised and expanded ed.). Kathmandu, Nepal: Centre for Development Studies.

New Spotlight. (2014). Sustainable agriculture: INGOs join hands. *New Spotlight, 8*(4). Retrieved August 20, 2015, from www.spotlightnepal.com/News/Article/SUSTAINABLE-AGRICULTURE-INGOs-Join-Hands

Nikku, B. R. (2010a). Social work education and practice in Nepal: Perspectives for internationalisation and indigenisation. In E. P. Eyebiyi, P. Herrmann, & V. Sheen (Eds.), *Global crossroads in social welfare: Emergent issues, debates and innovations across the globe* (Vol. 11, pp. 95–112). Bremen, Germany: Europaischer Hochschulverlag GmbH & Co.

Nikku, B. R. (2010b). Social work education in Nepal: Major opportunities and abundant challenges. *Social Work Education, 29*(8), 818–830. doi:10.1080/02615479.2010.5 16984

Nikku, B. R. (2013). Social work education in South Asia: A Nepalese perspective. In C. Noble, M. Henrickson, & I. Y. Han (Eds.), *Social work education: Voices from the Asia Pacific* (pp. 227–244). Sydney, NSW: Sydney University Press.

Nikku, B. R. (2014). Social work education in South Asia: Diverse, dynamic and disjointed? In C. Noble, H. Strauss, & B. Littlechild (Eds.), *Global social work: Crossing borders, blurring boundaries* (pp. 97–112). Sydney, NSW: Sydney University Press.

Nikku, B. R. (2015). Living through and responding to disasters: Multiple roles for social work. *Social Work Education, 34*(6), 601–606.

Nikku, B. R., Udas, P. B., & Adhikari, D. R. (2014). Grassroots innovations in social work teaching and learning: Case of Nepal School of Social Work. In B. R. Nikku & Z. A. Hatta (Eds.), *Social work education and practice: Scholarship and innovation in the Asia Pacific* (pp. 35–53). Sydney, NSW: Primrose Hall Publishing Group.

Nikolov, P. (2009). *International NGO peacebuilding: How INGOs facilitate Nepal's transition to peace.* Department of Political Science, Lund University. Retrieved December 15, 2015, from http://lup.lub.lu.se/luur/download?func=downloadFile&recordOId=1524582&fileOId=1551164

Nimmagadda, J., & Balgopal, P. R. (2000). Indigenisation of social work knowledge: An exploration of the process. *Asia Pacific Journal of Social Work, 10*(2), 4–18.

Nimmagadda, J., & Chakradhar, K. (2006). Indigenization of AA in South India. *Asia Pacific Journal of Social Work, 16*(1), 7–20.

Nimmagadda, J., & Cowger, C. (1999). Cross cultural practice: Social worker ingenuity in the indigenisation of practice knowledge. *International Social Work, 42*(3), 261–276.

Nimmagadda, J., & Martell, D. R. (2008). Home-made social work: The two-way transfer of social work practice knowledge between India and the USA. In M. Gray, J. Coates, & M. Yellow Bird (Eds.), *Indigenous social work around the world: Towards culturally relevant education and practice* (pp. 153–164). Aldershot, Hants: Ashgate.

Nozick, R. (2013). *Anarchy, state, and utopia.* New York, NY: Basic Books.

O'Connor, A. (2002). Poverty in global terms. In V. Desai & R. B. Potter (Eds.), *The companion to development studies* (pp. 37–41). London: Arnold.

O'Donnell, G. A., Cullel, J. V., & Iazzetta, O. M. (Eds.). (2004). *The quality of democracy: Theory and applications.* Notre Dame, IN: University of Notre Dame Press.

Oldfield, N. A. (1880). *Sketches from Nepal.* London: Allen and Company.

Onta, P., & Katherine, D. C. (2004). *Nepal ko sandarva ma samaj shastriya chintan* [Social scientific thinking in the context of Nepal]. Kathmandu, Nepal: Social Science Baha Himal Association.

Osei-Hwedie, K. (1993). The challenge of social work in Africa: Starting the indigenization. *Journal of Social Development in Africa, 8*(1), 19–30.

Osei-Hwedie, K. (1996). *The indigenization of social work practice and education: Vision or vanity?* Inaugural Lecture, University of Botswana, September 25.

Osei-Hwedie, K. (2002). Indigenous practice-some informed guesses: Self-evident and possible. *Social Work-Stellenbosch, 38*(4), 311–323.

Osei-Hwedie, K., & Rankopo, M. J. (2008). Developing culturally relevant social work education in Africa: The case of Botswana. In M. Gray, J. Coates, & M. Yellow Bird (Eds.), *Indigenous social work around the world: Towards culturally relevant education and practice* (pp. 203–218). Aldershot, Hants: Ashgate.

Panday, D. R. (1999). *Nepal's failed development: Reflections on the mission and the maladies.* Kathmandu, Nepal: Nepal South Asia Centre.

Panday, D. R. (2011). *Looking at development and donors: Essays from Nepal.* Kathmandu, Nepal: Martin Chautari.

Panday, D. R. (2012). The legacy of Nepal's failed development. In S. von Einsiedel, D. M. Malone, & S. Pradhan (Eds.), *Nepal in transition: From people's war to fragile peace* (pp. 81–99). New Delhi, India: Cambridge University Press.

Pandey, J. P., Dhakal, M. R., Karki, S., Poudel, P., & Pradhan, M. S. (2013). *Maternal and child health in Nepal: The effects of caste, ethnicity, and regional identity: Further analysis of the*

2011 Nepal demographic and health survey. Calverton, MD, USA: Nepal Ministry of Health and Population, New ERA and ICF International.

Parajuli, M. N., Luitel, C., Upreti, B. R., Gautam, P. R., Bhandari, B. K., Dhakal, R. K., & Munakarmi, R. (2015). *Nepali society and development: Relevance of the Nordic model in Nepal*. Kathmandu, Nepal: Royal Norwegian Embassy.

Patel, L. (2005). *Social welfare and social development in South Africa*. Cape Town, South Africa: Oxford University Press.

Patel, L., & Hochfeld, T. (2012). Developmental social work in South Africa: Translating policy into practice. *International Social Work, 56*(5), 690–704.

Pawar, M., & Tsui, M.-S. (2012). Social work in Southern and Eastern Asia. In K. Lyons, T. Hokenstad, M. Pawar, N. Huegler, & N. Hall (Eds.), *The Sage handbook of international social work* (pp. 407–420). Thousand Oaks, CA: Sage Publications.

Payne, M. (1997). *Modern social work theory* (2nd ed.). Basingstoke, Hants: Palgrave Macmillan.

Payne, M. (2005). *Modern social work theory* (3rd ed.). Basingstoke, Hants: Palgrave Macmillan.

Pelz, W. (2014). *The scope of understanding in sociology*. Hoboken, NJ: Taylor & Francis.

Pfaff-Czarnecka, J. (2004a). High expectations, deep disappointment: Politics, state and society in Nepal after 1990. In M. Hutt (Ed.), *Himalayan people's war: Nepal's Maoist revolution* (pp. 166–191). Bloomington, IN: Indiana University Press.

Pfaff-Czarnecka, J. (2004b). Vestiges and visions: Cultural change in the process of nation-building in Nepal. In D. N. Gellner, J. Pfaff-Czarnecka, & J. Whelpton (Eds.), *Nationalism and ethnicity in a Hindu kingdom: The politics of culture in contemporary Nepal* (pp. 419–472). New York, NY: Routledge.

Pfaff-Czarnecka, J. (2008). Distributional coalitions in Nepal: An essay on democratization, capture, and (lack of) confidence. In D. N. Gellener & K. Hatchethu (Eds.), *Governance, conflict and civic action series* (Vol. 1, pp. 71–104). New Delhi, India: Sage Publications.

Piety, M. G. (2010). *Ways of knowing: Kierkegaard's pluralist epistemology*. Waco, TX: Baylor University Press.

Pigg, S. L. (1992). Inventing social categories through place: Social representations and development in Nepal. *Comparative Studies of South Asia, Africa and the Middle East, 34*(3), 491–513.

Pigg, S. L. (1993). Unintended consequences: The ideological impact of development in Nepal. *Comparative Studies of South Asia, Africa and the Middle East, 13*(1&2), 45–47.

Pinderhuges, E. (1979). Teaching empathy in cross-cultural social work. *Social Work, 24*(4), 312–316. doi:10.1093/sw/24.4.312

Pinderhuges, E. (1984). Teaching empathy: Ethnicity, race and power and the crosscultural treatment interface. *American Journal of Social Psychiatry, 4*, 5–12.

Portes, A. (1997). Neoliberalism and the sociology of development: Emerging trends and unanticipated facts. *Population and Development Review, 23*(2), 229–259.

Powell, F. W. (2001). *The politics of social work*. London: Sage Publications.

Pradhan, K. (1991). *The Gorkha conquests: The process and consequences of the unification of Nepal, with particular reference to Eastern Nepal*. Calcutta, India: Oxford University Press.

Pugh, R., & Gould, N. (2000). Globalization, social work and social welfare. *European Journal of Social Work, 3*(2), 123–138.

Pumphrey, M. W. (1956). *Mary Richmond and the rise of professional social work in Baltimore: The foundations of a creative career*. New York, NY: Columbia University Press.

Putnam, R. D., Leonardi, R., & Nanetti, R. Y. (1994). *Making democracy work: Civic traditions in modern Italy*. Princeton, NJ: Princeton University Press.

Ragab, I. A. (1982). *Authenitisation of social work in developing countries*. Tanta, Egypt: Integrated Social Service Project.

Ragab, I. A. (1990). How social work can take root in developing countries. *Social Development Issues, 12*(3), 38–51.

Ragab, I. A. (1995). Middle East and Egypt. In T. D. Watts, D. Elliott, & N. S. Mayadas (Eds.), *International handbook on social work education* (pp. 281–304). Westport, CT: Greenwood Press.

Ragab, I. A. (2017). Has social work come of age? Revisiting the authentisation debate 25 years on. In M. Gray (Ed.), *Routledge handbook of social work and social development in Africa* (pp. 33–45). London: Routledge.

Rankin, K. N. (2001). Governing development: Neoliberalism, microcredit, and rational economic woman. *Economy and Society, 30*(1), 18–37.

Rao, J. (2010). The caste system: Effects on poverty in India, Nepal, and Sri Lanka. *Global Majority, 1*(2), 97–106.

Rao, V. (2012). Political context of social work. *Indian Journal of Dalit and Tribal Social Work, 1*(2), 14–34.

Rao, V. (2013). Decolonizing social work: An Indian view point. In M. Gray, J. Coates, M. Yellow Bird, & T. Hetherington (Eds.), *Decolonizing social work* (pp. 43–62). Aldershot, Hants: Ashgate.

Rawls, J. (2009). *A theory of justice*. Cambridge, MA: Harvard University Press.

Regmi, M. C. (1976). *Landownership in Nepal*. Los Angeles, CA: University of California Press.

Regmi, M. P. (1997). Nepal. In G. A. Postiglione & G. C. L. Mak (Eds.), *Asian higher education: An international handbook and reference guide* (pp. 217–230). Westport, CT: Greenwood Press.

Resnick, R. P. (1976). Conscientization: An indigenous approach to international social work. *International Social Work, 19*(2), 21–29.

Resnick, R. P. (1995). South America. In T. D. Watts, D. Elliott, & N. S. Mayadas (Eds.), *International handbook on social work education* (pp. 65–85). Westport, CT: Greenwood Press.

Riaz, A., & Basu, S. (2010). *Paradise lost? State failure in Nepal*. New York, NY: Roman & Littlefield Publisher, Inc.

Richmond, M. E. (1907). *The good neighbor in the modern city*. Philadelphia, PA: J. B. Lippincott Company.

Rigney, L.-I. (1999). Internationalization of an indigenous anticolonial cultural critique of research methodologies: A guide to indigenist research methodology and its principles. *Wicazo Sa Review, 14*(2), 109–121. doi:10.2307/1409555

Ritchie, J., & Rau, C. (2010). Kia mau ki te wairuatanga: Counter narratives of early childhood education in Aotearoa. In G. S. Cannella & L. D. Soto (Eds.), *Childhood: A handbook* (pp. 355–373). New York, NY: Peter Lang.

Robertson, D. (1993). *The Penguin dictionary of politics*. London: Penguin Books.

Robertson, R. (1992). *Globalization: Social theory and global culture*. Thousand Oaks, CA: Sage Publications.

Robertson, R. (1994). Globalisation or glocalisation? *The Journal of International Communication, 1*(1), 33–52. doi:10.1080/13216597.1994.9751780

Robinson, M. (1994). Governance, democracy and conditionality: NGOs and the new policy agenda. In A. Clayton (Ed.), *Governance, democracy and conditionality: What role for NGOs?* (pp. 35–51). Oxford, UK: INTRAC.

Rose, L. E. (1969). Regional development in South Asia: Nepal's role and attitude. In S. P. Varma & K. P. Misra (Eds.), *Foreign policies in South Asia* (pp. 356–364). Bombay, India: Orient Longman.

Rotberg, R. I. (2003). Failed states, collapsed states, weak states: Cause and indicators. In R. I. Rotberg (Ed.), *State failure and state weakness in a time of terror* (pp. 1–25). Washington, DC: Brookings Institution Press.

Rotberg, R. I. (2010). The failure and collapse of nation-states: Breakdown, prevention, and repair. In R. I. Rotberg (Ed.), *When states fail: Causes and consequences* (pp. 1–50). Princeton, NJ: Princeton University Press.

Rousseau, J. J. (1968). *The social contract*. London: Penguin Books.

Salamon, L. M., & Anheir, H. K. (1997). Toward a common definition. In L. M. Salamon & H. K. Anheir (Eds.), *Defining the nonprofit sector: A cross-national analysis* (pp. 29–50). Manchester: Manchester University Press.

Sarantakos, S. (2005). *Social research* (3rd ed.). New York, NY: Palgrave Macmillan.

Savada, A. M. (1991). *Nepal: A country study*. Washington, DC: Library of Congress.

Savada, A. M. (1993). *Nepal and Bhutan: Country studies*. Washington, DC: Federal Research Division, Library of Congress.

Schepers, D. H. (2006). The impact of NGO network conflict on the corporate social responsibility strategies of multinational corporations. *Business & Society, 45*(3), 282–299.

Schlesinger, E. G., & Devore, W. (1995). Ethnic sensitive social work practice: The state of art. *Journal of Sociology and Social Welfare, 22*(1), 29–58.

Schock, K. (1999). People power and political opportunities: Social movement mobilization and outcomes in the Philippines and Burma. *Social Problems, 46*(3), 355–375. doi:10.2307/3097105

Schock, K. (2005). *Unarmed insurrections: People power movements in nondemocracies*. Minneapolis, MN: University of Minnesota Press.

Seidman, I. (2013). *Interviewing as qualitative research: A guide for researchers in education and the social sciences* (4th ed.). New York, NY: Teachers College Press.

Sen, A. (2011). *The idea of justice*. Cambridge, MA: Harvard University Press.

Shah, S. (1993). Throes of a fledgling nation. *Himal, 6*(2), 7–10.

Shah, S. (2008). *Civil society in uncivil place: Soft state and regime change in Nepal*. Washington, DC: Washington East-West Center.

Shakya, S. (2012). Unleashing Nepal's economic potential: A business perspective. In S. von Einsiedel, D. M. Malone, & S. Pradhan (Eds.), *Nepal in transition: From people's war to fragile peace* (pp. 114–128). New Delhi, India: Cambridge University Press.

Sharma, K. L. (1997). *Social stratification in India: Issues and themes*. New Delhi, India: Sage Publications.

Shawky, A. (1972). Social work education in Africa. *International Social Work, 15*(1), 3–16.

Shrestha, N. P., Manandhar, H. K., Joshi, B. R., Sherchan, D. P., Paudel, K. P., Pradhan, A., & Gurung, T. B. (2008). Poverty alleviation through agriculture and rural development in Nepal. In J. W. Taco Bottema, G. Thompson, I. Wayan Rusastra, & R. Baldwin (Eds.), *Towards a joint regional agenda for the alleviation of poverty through agriculture and secondary crop development* (pp. 97–118). CAPSA Monograph No. 50. Retrieved December 15, 2015, from www.academia.edu/4091938/Towards_a_Joint_Regional_Agendafor_the_Alleviation_of_Poverty_through_Agriculture_and_Secondary_Crop_Development

Shrestha, N. R. (1997). *In the name of development: A reflection on Nepal*. New York, NY: University Press of America.

Shrestha, N. R. (2000). Book Review [Review of the book Nepal's failed development: Reflections on the mission and the maladies by Panday D. R.]. *Comparative Studies of South Asia, Africa and the Middle East, 20*(1&2), 154–155.

Shrestha, N. R. (2002). *Nepal and Bangladesh: A global studies handbook.* Santa Barbara, CA: ABC-CLIO.

Shrestha, N. R., & Bhattrai, K. (2017). *Historical dictionary of Nepal* (2nd ed.). Lanham, MD: Rowman and Littlefield.

Shrestha, S. K. (2013). *History of social work in Nepal.* Kathmandu, Nepal: University Grant Commission.

Sill, M., & Kirkby, J. (2013). *Atlas of Nepal in the modern world.* New York, NY: Earthscan.

Sinclair, R. (2004). Aboriginal social work education in Canada: Decolonizing pedagogy for the seventh generation. *First People Child and Family Review, 1*(1), 49–61.

Sinclair, R., & Albert, J. (2008). Social work and the anti-oppressive stance: Does the emperor really have new clothes? *Critical Social Work, 9*(1).

Sinclair, R., Hart, M. A., & Bruyere, G. (Eds.). (2009). *Wicihitowin: Aboriginal social work in Canada.* Halifax, NS: Fernwood Publishing.

Singh, M. P., & Kukreja, V. (2014). *Federalism in South Asia.* London: Routledge.

Smith, L. T. (1999). *Decolonising methodologies: Research and indigenous peoples.* London: Zed Books.

Smith, L. T. (2012). *Decolonising methodologies: Research and indigenous peoples* (2nd ed.). London: Zed Books.

Social Welfare Council. (2014a). *Brief information of INGOs working under agreement with Social Welfare Council (FY 2070/071).* Kathmandu, Nepal: SWC. Retrieved April 21, 2015, from www.swc.org.np/SWC%20rel%20Doc/INGOs%20Detail%20Information%202070_071.pdf

Social Welfare Council. (2014b). *SWC Sectorwise NGOs.* Retrieved April 19, 2015, from www.swc.org.np/sectorwisengo_list.php

Social Welfare Council. (2015a). *List of INGOs working under agreement with Social Welfare Council.* Retrieved December 7, 2015, from www.swc.org.np/wp-content/uploads/2015/06/List-of-INGOs-2071_72.pdf

Social Welfare Council. (2015b). *NGOs affiliated with Social Welfare Council.* Retrieved December 7, 2015, from www.swc.org.np/wp-content/uploads/2015/08/SWC_NGOs_2034_071-asadh.pdf

Social Work Institute. (2013). *About us.* Retrieved May 12, 2014, from www.swi-nepal.org/eng/detail_about_us.php

Soja, E. (1989). *Postmodern geographies: The reassertion of space in critical social theory.* New York, NY: Verso.

Somers, M. R. (1994). The narrative constitution of identity: A relational and network approach. *Theory and Society, 23*(5), 605–649.

Spair, P., & Moser, C. (2007). *International NGOs and poverty reduction strategies: The contribution of an asset-based approach: Brookings global economy and development working paper 8.* Washington, DC: Brookings Institution Press.

Specht, H., & Courtney, M. E. (1994). *Unfaithful angels: How social work has abandoned it mission.* New York, NY: Free Press.

Spivak, G. C. (1999). *A critique of postcolonial reason: Toward a history of the vanishing present.* Cambridge, MA: Harvard University Press.

Srinivas, M. N. (1956). A not on Sanskritization and westernization. *The Far Eastern Quarterly, 15*(4), 481–496.

Stevens, S. F. (1996). *Claiming the high ground: Sherpas, subsistence, and environmental change in the highest Himalaya.* New Delhi, India: Motilal Banarsidass.

Strauss, A., & Corbin, J. (1990). *Basics of qualitative research: Grounded theory procedures and techniques*. Thousand Oaks, CA: Sage.

Strug, D. (2006). Community‑oriented social work in Cuba: Government response to emerging social problems. *Social Work Education, 25*(7), 749–762.

Tamburro, A. (2013). Including decolonisation in social work education and practice. *Journal of Indigenous Social Development, 2*(1), 1–16.

Tanaka, M. (2011). The changing roles of NGOs in Nepal: Promoting emerging rights-holder organizations for inclusive aid. *International Journal of Voluntary and Nonprofit Organizations, 22*(3), 494–517. doi:10.1007/s11266-010-9173-1

Taylor, G. (2012). State department drops Maoists from terrorist watch list. *The Washington Times*. Retrieved January 12, 2014, from www.washingtontimes.com/news/2012/sep/6/us-removes-nepal-communists-from-terrorist-list/

Tejeda, C., Espinoza, M., & Gutierrez, K. (2003). Toward a decolonzing pedagogy: Social justice reconsidered. In P. P. Trifonas (Ed.), *Pedagogy of difference: Rethinking education for social change* (pp. 10–37). New York, NY: RoutledgeFalmer.

Temple, D. (1997). NGOs: A trojan horse. In M. Rahnema & V. Bawtree (Eds.), *The post-development reader* (pp. 202–203). London: Zed Books.

Thapa, D. (2012). The making of Maoist insurgency. In S. von Einsiedel, D. M. Malone, & S. Pradhan (Eds.), *Nepal in transition: From people's war to fragile peace* (pp. 37–57). New Delhi, India: Cambridge University Press.

Thapa, M. (2007). *Forget Kathmandu: An elegy for democracy*. London: Penguin Books.

Thieme, S., Bhattrai, R., Gurung, G., Kollmair, M., Manandhar, S., & Müller-Böker, U. (2005). Addressing the needs of Nepalese migrant workers in Nepal and in Delhi, India. *Mountain Research and Development, 25*(2), 109–114. doi:10.230 7/3674669

Thomas, G. M. (2007). The culture and religious character of world society. In P. Beyer & L. Beaman (Eds.), *Religion, globalization, and culture* (pp. 35–56). Boston, MA: Brill.

Tibaijuko, A. (2007, August 12–18). Keynote address on water for thirsty cities. World Water Week, Stockholm, Sweden.

Tilly, C. (1975). Reflections on the history of European state-making. In C. Tilly (Ed.), *The formation of national states in western Europe* (pp. 3–84). Princeton, NJ: Princeton University Press.

Tilly, C. (1985). War making and state making as organized crime. In P. Evans, D. Reuschmeyer, & T. Skocpol (Eds.), *Bringing the state back in* (pp. 169–191). Cambridge, MA: Cambridge University Press.

Transparency International. (2014). *Corruption perceptions index 2014*. Berlin, Germany: Transparency International.

Tsang, A. K. T., & Yan, M.-C. (2001). Chinese corpus, western application: The Chinese strategy of engagement with western social work discourse. *International Social Work, 44*(4), 433–454. doi:10.1177/002087280104400404

United Nations Development Program. (1994). *Human development report 1994: New dimensions of human society*. New York, NY: UNDP.

United Nations Development Program. (2009). *Nepal human development report 2009*. Kathmandu, Nepal: UNDP.

United Nations Development Program. (2013). *Human development report 2013: The rise of the south: Human progress in a diverse world*. New York, NY: UNDP.

United Nations Development Program. (2014a). *Human development report 2014: Sustaining human progress: Reducing vulnerabilities and building resilience*. New York, NY: UNDP.

United Nations Development Program. (2014b). *Nepal annual report*. Kathmandu, Nepal: UNDP.

United Nations International Children Emergency Fund. (2013). *State of the world's children: Nepal*. Retrieved November 25, 2015, from www.unicef.org/infobycountry/nepal_nepal_statistics.html

United Nations International Children Emergency Fund. (2015). *Nepal earthquake: Update*. Retrieved September 24, 2015, from www.unicef.or.th/ supportus/content/nepal-earthquake-unicef-responds

United Nations, International Monetary Fund, European Commission, World Bank, & Organization for Economic Co-operation and Development. (2009). *System of national accounts*. New York, NY: UN, IMF, EC, WB, and OECD.

United Nations Nepal. (2013). *Nepal: Constituent assembly election 2013 under FPTP: Breakdown of elected candidates by caste/ethnicity*. Retrieved December 29, 2015, from http://un.org.np/maps/nepal-constituent-assembly-election-2013-under-fptp-breakdown-elected-candidates-casteethnicity

University Grant Commission. (2011). *Education management information system/report on higher education 2010/11*. Kathmandu, Nepal: University Grant Commission.

Uvin, P. (1998). *Aiding violence: The development enterprise in Rwanda*. West Hartford, CT: Kumarian Press.

Vaidya, T. R. (1993). *Prithvinarayan Shah, the founder of modern Nepal*. New Delhi, India: Anmol Publications.

Van Lookcke, J. H., & Philipson, L. (2002). *Report of the European Commission on conflict prevention assessment mission*. Kathmandu, Nepal: European Union Commission.

Vikala, R. (2000). *A leaf in a begging bowl: Modern Nepali stories* (M. Thapa, Trans.). Kathmandu, Nepal: Mandala Book Point.

von Einsiedel, S., Malone, D. M., & Pradhan, S. (2012a). Introduction. In S. von Einsiedel, D. M. Malone, & S. Pradhan (Eds.), *Nepal in transition: From people's war to fragile peace* (pp. 1–36). New Delhi, India: Cambridge University Press.

von Einsiedel, S., Malone, D. M., & Pradhan, S. (Eds.). (2012b). *Nepal in transition: From people's war to fragile peace*. New Delhi, India: Cambridge University Press.

Wallensteen, P. (2014). Theoretical developments in understanding the origins of civil war. In E. Newman & K. DeRouen (Eds.), *Routledge handbook of civil wars* (pp. 13–27). London: Taylor & Francis.

Walton, R. G., & Nasr, M. M. A. E. (1988). Indigenisation and authentisation in terms of social work in Egypt. *International Social Work*, *31*(1), 135–144.

Waterfall, B. F. (2002). Native people and the social work profession: A critical exploration of colonising problematics and the development of decolonised thought. *Journal of Educational Thought*, *36*(2), 149–166.

Waterfall, B. F. (2008). *Decolonizing Anishnabec social work education: An Anishnabe spiritually-infused reflexive study*. Toronto, ON: University of Toronto Press.

Weaver, H. N. (1998). Indigenous people in a multicultural society: Unique issues for human services. *Social Work*, *43*(3), 203–211.

Weaver, H. N. (1999). Indigenous people and the social work profession: Defining culturally competent services. *Social Work*, *44*(3), 217–225.

Weaver, H. N. (2008). Indigenous social work in the united States: Reflections on Indian Tacos, Trojan horse and Canoes filled with indigenous revolutionaries. In M. Gray, J. Coates, & M. Yellow Bird (Eds.), *Indigenous social work around the world: Towards culturally relevant education and practice* (pp. 71–81). Aldershot, Hants: Ashgate.

Webb, S. A. (2003). Local orders and global chaos in social work. *European Journal of Social Work*, *6*(2), 191–204.

Weisbord, B. A. (1988). *The non-profit economy*. Cambridge, MA: Harvard University Press.

Whelpton, J. (2005). *A history of Nepal*. Cambridge, MA: Cambridge University Press.

Wilmer, F. (1993). *The indigenous voice in the world politics*. Thousand Oaks, CA: Sage Publications.

Wilson, S. (2013). Using indigenist research to shape our future. In M. Gray, J. Coates, M. Yellow Bird, & T. Hetherington (Eds.), *Decolonizing social work* (pp. 311–322). Aldershot, Hants: Ashgate.

Wong, Y.-L. R. (2002). Reclaiming Chinese women's subjectivities: Indigenizing "social work with women" in China through postcolonial ethnography. *Women's Studies International Forum, 25*(1), 67–77.

World Bank. (2003). *Financial accountability in Nepal: Country assessment*. Washington, DC: World Bank.

World Bank. (2018). *Country profile: Nepal*. Retrieved from http://databank.worldbank.org/data/views/reports/reportwidget.aspx?Report_Name=CountryProfile&Id=b450fd57&tbar=y&dd=y&inf=n&zm=n&country=NPL

World Health Organization Commission on the Social Determinants of Health. (2008). *Closing the gap in a generation: Health equity through action on the social determinants of health*. Geneva, Switzerland: WHO.

Yadav, R. K. (2016). Social work(ers) in nation building. In P. Jaiswal (Ed.), *Understanding Nepal in contemporary times* (pp. 245–272). New Delhi, India: Synergy.

Yan, M.-C., & Cheung, K. W. (2006). The politics of indigenization: A case study of development of social work in China. *Journal of Sociology and Social Welfare, 33*(2), 63–83.

Yan, M.-C., & Tsui, M.-S. (2007). The quest for western social work knowledge: Literature in the USA and practice in China. *International Social Work, 50*(5), 641–653.

Yang, K. S. (1995). Chinese social orientation: An integrative analysis. In T. Y. Lin, W. S. Tseng, & E. K. Yeh (Eds.), *Chinese societies and mental health* (pp. 19–39). Hong Kong: Oxford University Press.

Yellow Bird, M. (2008). Terms of endearment: A brief dictionary for decolonizing social work with indigenous peoples. In M. Gray, J. Coates, & M. Yellow Bird (Eds.), *Indigenous social work around the world: Towards culturally relevant education and practice* (pp. 275–291). Aldershot, Hants: Ashgate.

Yellow Bird, M. (2013). Neurodecolonization: Applying mindfulness research to decolonizing social work. In M. Gray, J. Coates, M. Yellow Bird, & T. Hetherington (Eds.), *Decolonizing social work* (pp. 293–310). Aldershot, Hants: Ashgate.

Yip, K.-S. (2002). Transcendence from trauma and terrorism: A Taoistic reflection. *Families in Society: The Journal of Contemporary Human Services, 83*(4), 403–404.

Yip, K.-S. (2005a). A dynamic Asian response to globalisation in cross-cultural social work. *International Social Work, 48*(5), 593–607.

Yip, K.-S. (2005b). Chinese concepts of mental health: Cultural implication for social work practice. *International Social Work, 48*(4), 391–407.

Young, I. M. (2009). Five faces of oppression. In G. Henderson & M. Waterstone (Eds.), *Geographic thoughts: A praxis perspective* (pp. 55–71). London: Routledge.

Yunong, H., & Xiong, Z. (2008). A reflection on the indigenization discourse in social work. *International Social Work, 51*(5), 611–622.

Zoabi, K., & Savaya, R. (2012). Cultural intervention strategies employed by Arab social workers in Israel: Identification and conceptualisation. *British Journal of Social Work, 42*(2), 245–264. doi:10.1093/bjsw/bcr071

Zunes, S. (1994). Unarmed insurrections against authoritarian governments in the Third World: A new kind of revolution. *Third World Quarterly, 15*(3), 403–426.

Index

Note: Page numbers in italics indicate a figure and page numbers in bold indicate a table on the corresponding page.

Milton Keynes UK
Ingram Content Group UK Ltd.
UKHW040057071024
449327UK00019B/612

9 780367 671471